The Psychotherapy
of the Self

The Psychotherapy
of the Self

By

Hyman L. Muslin, M.D.
and
Eduardo R. Val, M.D.

BRUNNER/MAZEL *Publishers* • New York

We gratefully acknowledge permission to reprint the following passages that appear in Chapter 7:

Gitelson, M. (1952). The emotional position of the analyst in the psychoanalytic situation. *International Journal of Psycho-Analysis, 33*, pp. 6–7.
Kohut, H. (1971). *Analysis of the self* (pp. 287–288). New York: International Universities Press.
Tower, L. (1956). Countertransference. *Journal of the American Psychoanalytic Association, 4*, pp. 27–28.

Library of Congress Cataloging-in-Publication Data

Muslin, Hyman L., 1929–
  The psychotherapy of the self.

  Bibliography: p. 209
  Includes index.
  1. Self. 2. Psychotherapy. I. Val, Eduardo R.
II. Title. [DNLM: 1. Ego. 2. Psychoanalytic Therapy.
3. Psychotherapy. WM 420 M987p]
RC489.S43M87 1987   616.89′14   87–6356
ISBN 0-87630-464-1

Copyright © 1987 by Hyman L. Muslin and Eduardo R. Val

Published by
BRUNNER/MAZEL, INC.
19 Union Square
New York, New York 10003

MANUFACTURED IN THE UNITED STATES OF AMERICA

10 9 8 7 6 5 4 3 2 1

Foreword

When the writings of Heinz Kohut first appeared they were clearly and recognizably directed to a psychoanalytic audience. The initial papers and his first book were modest in their scope and were meant primarily to direct the attention of psychoanalysts to a subgroup of personality pathology, i.e., the narcissistic personality disorders. For the most part, the reception to the ideas was cordial and even enthusiastic, since it seemed to be a significant expansion of the extant body of psychoanalytic knowledge. The objective observer of the scientific community of psychoanalysis could only be impressed by this open embracing of new concepts. As the writing of Kohut became a bit more daring and looked like it was covering more territory that had been under the aegis of what came to be called classical psychoanalysis, a certain note of caution and concern began to be heard in the same community of scholars. This warning began to carry a somewhat shrill tone of negativism in its message, and, amidst the many criticisms levelled against what came to be called self psychology, was the one that said it was fundamentally not psychoanalysis but psychotherapy. Now usually that pronouncement is made after one or two prefatory sentences or paragraphs that claim that there is certainly nothing wrong with psychotherapy and lots of people need and benefit from it, but a note of condescension and disdain always seems to creep into the final dispatch of self psychology into the land of psychotherapy: one which is a rather large and uneven and poorly regulated principality that lies in proximity to the kingdom of analysis.

One of the biggest problems in the effort to segregate psychoanalysis from psychotherapy and then to assign self psychology to that domain was that no one knew for sure just what analysis was, and even fewer (if that is possible) could tell us what psychotherapy was. The difference between these two ill-defined and amorphous arenas did, however, seem to hinge on one principle point: psychotherapy was less than psychoanalysis, either a dilution or a fraction or a superficiality. You saw the patient less, you used less furniture, you might even charge less, but to make up for these deficiencies you were allowed to talk a little more. Amidst all of the efforts to derive psychotherapy from psychoanalysis there seemed a rather clear lack of a solid theoretical base on which one could stand to clearly spell out the distinctions.

The same observer of the psychoanalytic community during the introduction and growing influence of self psychology would also have observed the enormous popularity of the writings of Kohut and others amongst what came to be called nonanalysts. There is no doubt that the vast majority of therapy in this country is conducted by mental health professionals who are not psychiatrists and/or are not trained in institutes sanctioned by the American Psychoanalytic Association. It is easy to dismiss these therapists as undertrained and ill-qualified, but they probably have the same percentages of brilliant and mediocre practitioners as any group. The social phenomenon that arose with this heterogeneous group that practices most psychotherapy was an enthusiastic, some might say overenthusiastic, interest and investment in self psychology. At last there seemed to be a theory that made sense of what many of these clinicians had been doing or had tried to do in their professional lives. Of course, this heightened involvement in self psychology by psychotherapists served to reinforce the charge of "this is not analysis" that was directed toward the enthusiasts of self psychology. But it slowly became clear that the theory behind psychoanalytic self psychology could lend a framework to the range of activities that covers both psychoanalysis and psychotherapy. And now we have a book that demonstrates it!

The authors of this monograph modestly set out to sketch the theory of self psychology that explains the three divisions of treatment: supportive psychotherapy, uncovering psychotherapy, and psychoanalysis. I use the word "modest" because they write without any attempt to depreciate or argue against other books on psychotherapy which lean heavily on classical psychoanalysis. Nor do they warn the reader to stay away from dreams, or avoid transference interpretations or any of the host of injunctions used to keep analysis pure and often resulting in confusing or frightening psychotherapists. They rely on a number of illustrative cases to show what they do and how they do it. I must confess to a personal prejudice to explain why I so enjoyed these cases. I recently read another, somewhat similar book which relied heavily on case illustrations. Almost every other page had a clinical vignette, and I found it almost numbing. The patients were all different, and I always have a great deal of trouble getting to know a patient in a few paragraphs only to have a totally different one presented after a few pages. Muslin and Val rely on but a few cases, and they reintroduce them as they become relevant in succeeding chapters. I felt that I "knew" the patients well enough to rather easily become reacquainted with them in a different context. The authors are not only empathic with their patients but with their readers as well.

This is not just another book on psychotherapy. Nor is it but an effort toward a more digestible rehash of the tenets of self psychology. Rather it is a most needed marriage of the theory of self psychology with the activity of our therapeutic efforts. It gives both the novice and the veteran an opportunity to judge how psychoanalytic self psychology has grown up to the stature of explaining the varieties of all intervention from support to analysis. And like any good marriage, it is a cause for celebration.

Arnold Goldberg, M.D.

Contents

Preface

Several *considerations* have influenced the shape of and emphases in this volume. A major consideration has been our long-held wish to advance our view that psychotherapeutic treatment should be a planned effort based on carefully gathered data. From the data of the initial interviews the therapist is to establish a diagnosis of the patient's difficulties and plug in the appropriate therapy. The therapist, therefore, must become sufficiently versed in each of the major psychotherapeutic modalities, especially the goals of each of the therapeutic approaches.

Still another consideration in our work has been to present the therapeutic process in each of the therapeutic approaches by case examples. In this way the reader can see the data that recommend a particular modality, and then be with the therapist step-by-step as he or she executes the particular interventions associated with the therapeutic modality being used. We have introduced in each of the chapters on the particular therapies a description of the goals of each of the approaches, the methods by which these goals are reached, and the outcome results to be attained in each of the therapies.

Throughout this book, we have attempted to apply the teachings of Kohut's self psychology in understanding our patients' difficulties and in understanding their needs for resolution or alleviation of their distresses.

We have offered a special chapter on the development of the self and an understanding of psychopathology from the view of self psychology. We have also included a chapter on a topic that we know to be quite relevant for the psychotherapist: the inner world of the psychotherapist, which stresses his potentially interfering transferences and subjective reactions.

A final consideration throughout this book has been our attempt to look at the learning needs of the expert psychotherapist as well as the learning needs of the psychotherapist who is at an earlier stage of development. We hope that our endeavors to strike a balance have been realized.

A few words about the bibliography are in order, we believe. Our main intention in this book has been to present to the reader in the "flesh" a clinician at work, demonstrating the varied tasks of the therapist, his observation of data, his arrival at the empathic understanding guiding his diagnostic assessments and therapeutic interventions, while attempting to engage the reader in an author-reader alliance and involving the reader as a participant-observer. To that extent we purposely limited distracting the reader with unnecessary references or prolonged theoretical discussions—albeit useful in other contexts.

We acknowledge in the general bibliography those authors whose contributions have provided the basis for, or influenced our thinking and approaches throughout, this volume. In particular, we have included the work of self psychology authors, many of whom we have had the privilege of being in personal contact with over the years, whose ideas and dialogues made them silent and sharing partners throughout this volume.

In summing up our preface to this volume, we would stress that everyone in our field must become expert or proficient in: 1) data gathering and establishing a diagnosis of the specific self-distress; 2) ascertaining the goals and end results of the different psychotherapies; 3) plugging in or assigning the appropriate therapeutic modality in each case.

Acknowledgments

The authors wish to express their gratitude to several people who have been of service in the production of this book. We wish to offer our appreciation to our indispensable others, Bernice and Patricia and our children, Anthony, Suzanne and Elizabeth and Daniela, Gabriel and Sebastian. Their infusion of mirroring and soothing, as always, was vital to our cohesiveness. Our secretaries, Barbara Edwards and Marjorie Reinfoe, were of great help in the preparation of this volume.

A special note of gratitude is necessary to offer to Ann Alhadeff, our editor at Brunner/Mazel. She was consistently careful of our words and caretaking of our self-esteem so as to maintain our equilibrium throughout the preparation of this volume.

We are indebted to our students at the University of Illinois and the Chicago Institute for Psychoanalysis for their invaluable aid in working with us as we refined our views on the teaching and learning of psychotherapy. We are also grateful for the stimulation offered by the participants in the Self Psychology Workshops of the Chicago Institute for Psychoanalysis.

Finally, hovering around us was the spirit of Heinz Kohut, who once said to one of us: "We make our words. Our words make us."

The Psychotherapy
of the Self

1

An Introduction to the Work of Being a Psychotherapist

This volume will present a body of skills and knowledge which we deem essential in the work of psychotherapy, from the diagnostic phase to termination. Psychotherapy, in our view, is no longer to be perceived as a vaguely defined set of operations instituted for those persons in a state of psychic distress who do not fit the criteria for psychoanalysis. On the contrary, there are three major psychotherapeutic modalities, each with its own indications, goals, and methodologies. The three psychotherapeutic approaches are those of the supportive psychotherapies, the uncovering or psychoanalytic psychotherapies, and psychoanalysis.

The particular therapy that will ultimately be utilized is based on the diagnosis which becomes, as it must, the major determinant of the psychotherapeutic modality. In performing the diagnostic work, the clinician must, therefore, derive a body of data—cognitive and empathic—which is an accurate reflection of the patient's psyche at that time. The essential elements in arriving at the data base necessary for the diagnosis are basic listening and understanding skills and, of course, a working knowledge of the different psychotherapies.

3

LISTENING AND OBSERVING AS A WAY OF LIFE

The technical requirements for performing a diagnosis and for all psychotherapy work begin with the skill of listening: cognitive listening to details of the interview and empathic listening to capture the patient's inner or experiential life.

Cognitive Observations

The data derived from the cognitive observations can be organized into the verbal and nonverbal behaviors as well as the subjective reactions of the therapist. In the data derived from the study of the *verbal behaviors* are the observations of the associations which the patient makes. The study and evaluation of the associations include attention to the "fit" of the associations. Do the associations reveal concordance in their elements, i.e., does each segment flow logically into the next segment or is there a significant amount of disharmony or derailing in the verbal associations, which may reflect the presence of a thinking disorder? Other observations gleaned from the study of the verbal behaviors are the type of speech or word patterns, the frequency and rapidity or paucity and retardation of the verbal behavior, as well as the themes revealed in the verbal behavior.

The nonverbal behaviors can be divided into the study of the manifest emotions, the affects, and other nonverbal behaviors. The observer will be interested in the affects that are present in the patient's behaviors as well as their relevance or inappropriateness. The description of the patient's affects will include the revealed affects as well as their relevance, mobility or fixity, and depth or shallowness. The other nonverbal behaviors include those of gestures, gait, grooming, and postures.

The final assessment of the so-called cognitive observations is of the therapist's *subjective* responses to the patient and/or the patient's material. Does the therapist experience compassion or uneasiness or something akin to indifference or even boredom? These latter observations are valuable in several ways: 1) They serve to indicate the patient's modal impact on people; and 2) they may highlight unique responses to the patient in the therapist which the latter can become alerted to, monitor, and investigate so that such response will not interfere with the gathering of data. All these behaviors—the so-called cognitive behaviors—are observable through the interviewer's close attention to the material of the patient's responses.

It is important to set a tone early in one's interactions with the patient which indicates the interviewer's wish not to overtly respond to each of the patient's communications but rather to open up areas of thought and feeling to which the therapist will pay attention. The interviewer sets this tone by the following: 1) *abstinence* from segment-by-segment verbal responses to the patient's material in the interview; 2) *consonance*—the interviewer's responses when he or she does respond are in harmony with the patient's associations, rather than the interviewer directing the patient to new themes; 3) *nondirectiveness*—the interviewer by his evocative, nonspecific comments will endeavor to encourage the patient to describe his or her inner experiences and related thoughts and feelings (associations) rather than to center on detail.

Finally, in regard to cognitive observations, since the material here is manifest and therefore potentially observable, the observations must be capable of being *consensually validated*, i.e., every observer of the same material should be in substantial agreement about the verbal and nonverbal behaviors. These observations are findings—neither speculations nor subjective reactions—and they are to be reported as such; hence, "the affect was diminished . . . ," " . . . sad" or " . . . joyous." They should not be reported as, "In my view" or "I sense that such and such is going on" or "I have the feeling that the patient is experiencing such-and-such."

Empathy and Empathic Observations

Empathy is defined as a mode of observation that attempts to capture the subject's inner life, i.e., it is an attempt to know the intrapsychic or psychological in the observed subject. It requires, in the observer, the capacity to draw out of him/herself a self-state or experience that is thought to approximate that of the subject. Since empathic "observations" are surmises, they require validation in the form of supporting data from the patient's subsequent interview behaviors. The information that is gathered through empathy is, as noted, the whole of the self-experience. The therapist's attempts to place him/herself (through the process of vicarious introspection) in the patient's inner life and see the world from his side ultimately lead to the recognition of the current experience of the self. Thus, from the empathy view the patient is "observed" to be experiencing sadness or withdrawal, or is fragmented, or is immersed in ineptitude. These empathic observations may come after the therapist carefully gathers together the details of the cognitively observed behaviors; however, an empathic surmise is commonly made in reaction to a nonverbal behavior or a discrete comment (Basch, 1983a; Kohut, 1959; Muslin, 1974).

The importance of these empathic measurements lies in their being *the* major pathway to reaching the patient's inner life and to recognizing what he or she is experiencing from moment-to-moment in the sessions. Is the patient's experience of the world that of the youngster still in 1947 rather than 1987? The empathic assessments enable the therapist to know how the patient views his object-world. Is his experience of his current object world that he is surrounded by objects similar in every way to his childhood world of objects? These vital measurements of our patients enter into our baseline assessments; they tell us where our patients are located developmentally and therefore structurally, and thus how much has to be added to their selves to ensure cohesiveness. From the patient's side, the experience of being with someone whose sole intent is to understand one's inner life and not to engage in dialogue is a unique occurrence. Although it may ultimately be experienced as a positive and equilibrating force, it may at first be rejected out of the patient's fear of anticipated rejections to dependency.

The empathic assessments give the therapist the data to answer the initial query of the psychotherapy: *What* is the patient experiencing? The second query is: *Where* is (are) this (these) reaction(s) coming from? The final query in psychotherapy is: *What* is this reaction or self-state or defense or drive doing here *now*? These last two inquiries will be considered throughout this volume since they represent the basic questions that are to be illuminated in uncovering psychotherapy.

There are two areas of difficulty in empathic cognition: one is the capacity to initiate or maintain the use of empathic observations; the second is the accuracy of the empathic observations. The failure in initiation or maintenance is revealed in those observers whose capacity to make transient identifications (Fliess, 1942) is limited, so that their introspection (present self-experience) and empathy for themselves (past self-experience) are limited.

Kohut (1977) spoke of primary empathy failures, in which the subject was exposed to an unresponsive selfobject in childhood, the result being a person with little worth, whose self-strivings were repressed; thus the person could not genuinely recognize or appreciate the other's need in him/herself. These observers have very limited access to their inner mental life. They do not recognize in themselves, and therefore cannot in others, affect states, wishes for echo-approving, or needs for calming, since their narcissistic disappointments have resulted in permanent repressions and/or disavowals.

The second major empathic deficit lies in those whose capacity to sit in someone else's shoes is limited. Thus, although there may be the initiation of the empathic process, the empathy is inaccurate and the patient is not recognized for what *he* or *she* is experiencing. At times these empathic failures result from the absence in the observer of relevant self-memories that are similar to the observed subject—the difficulty in empathizing with people from grossly dissimilar economic, social, or gender circumstances (Muslin & Val, 1980). At other times, these empathic failures represent the phenomenon of transference onto a subject, so that the subject is perceived in harmony with the observer's needs rather than as he/she is in reality.

In sum, we have described the initial task of the psychotherapist to be the gatherer and observer of his patient from two vantage points: cognitive observations and empathic observations. We have further stated that an observer of the psyche learns early in our business that psychotherapeutic sessions—diagnostic as well as therapeutic—are *not* dialogues; rather, they are laboratories for careful and critical observations. Once this point is accepted, the therapist can focus his or her efforts on these cognitive and empathic tasks.

We previously alluded to the data-gathering principles of abstinence and consonance in psychotherapy work. *Abstinence,* as previously noted, refers to the principle that the patient is on center stage throughout our dealings with him, and that we abstain from dialogue—the mode of interaction in which each participant strives to appreciate the other. *Consonance,* to reemphasize, refers to the interviewer's or therapist's actions in making relevant or appropriate interactions in time (i.e., consonant) with the patient's material. It is based on the notion of associational listening, as well as the appreciation of the *essence* or essential aspect of the material under observation.

However, from the point of view of the therapist the essential task is that of *listening.* The therapist must train himself to listen to the moment-to-moment connections and the associated nonverbal material of affect and action connected with the word associations. Further, the therapist must train himself to sit in the patient's shoes, to become transiently merged with the subject rather than to become simply the object towards whom the patient is directing his comments. Becoming a lifelong listener is to be unimpeded by concerns such as the urge to "do" or "say" something. Those therapists who have understood this central task are concerned only about whether they were able to follow the details of the material, segment by segment, and were able to maintain an empathic posture throughout the entire session.

During the course of a diagnostic interview carefully followed, the therapist will need to clarify or illuminate certain details which are easily addressed within the context of the material that is being observed. We are not advocating silence; rather, we are advocating listening and observing as the central task of the psychotherapist, whether it is in the diagnostic or therapeutic phase of the work. Both clarification of questions in the diagnostic phase and interpretations in the therapy flow from the empathic and cognitive observations.

TRANSCRIPTS FROM A DIAGNOSTIC INTERVIEW

In the following examples, sequential transcripts from a diagnostic interview will be followed by the relevant cognitive and empathic observations.

The patient, Mr. M. S., was a tall, stately man who appeared to be in his fifties. He was neatly dressed but without a tie; the collar of his shirt stood out over his coat lapel. His demeanor was pleasant and there was a smile on his face as he related his difficulties. The pleasant appearance with the ever-present smile stood in contrast to the presenting complaints. They were as follows:

Segment 1

Therapist: Now, I know very little of you and your condition, so perhaps you could start from the beginning and tell me about yourself and your problems.

Mr. M. S.: Well, my problem right today is that I feel I'm a useless, unnecessary person and, er, I just don't want to go on living anymore. That's the way I feel. This is my whole problem. Er, I had a heart attack two years ago in March that kept me in the hospital for six weeks. Before that, I was having anginas for two or three years that I kept secret from the family. And after that I was in the hospital for four weeks and home for two weeks. Er, I went back to my work as a spotter—I'm in my own business now—I went back to work and was working for three months and then the man sold the business that I was working at and, er, I was unable to get a job after that and I didn't feel like working. I, er, worked part-time for about a year in a place, but the place was in chaos. I couldn't make any money and I quit that job and tried to get other jobs and was turned down and, er, felt absolutely inadequate to . . . to do anything anymore so I've just given up the desire or will, or whatever you want to call it, to just go on living. I feel inept, useless.

Observations

From the cognitive side, the verbal behavior revealed that the patient's associations fit together and were comprehensible. There was no difficulty in expression through words. The theme of this first segment was inferiority and uselessness connected with the heart attack he suffered. These experiences were also connected with his suicidal thoughts. The affect, however, was not that of mourning nor did his other nonverbal behaviors reveal a posture of dejection or agitation.

From the empathy side, the patient's comments revealed that he was immersed in the experience of a self without worth and therefore unable to comprehend much of any value in his life.

Segment 2

(The last comment by the patient was that he felt "useless")

Therapist: Since the heart attack?

Mr. M. S.: Since the heart attack. Before that, er, I had a good inflated ego. I was working and doing well . . . and did my work very well. I was a spotter in a cleaning plant for 30 years and I did my work well. Was well liked but after that the cleaning business has gone to pieces and now, I am . . . I feel inadequate to do anything else as far as working is concerned although I do have, what you call a, er, a knowledge of everything, a little knowledge of everything but complete knowledge of nothing, if you know what I mean. I'm a Johnny-come-lately. I could put a light in a sw . . . switch in a light, or I could do some carpenter work and I can put chains in windows and . . . and paint to an extent and hang wallpaper. Did all our own decorating all the time but now I'm just lazy. I have no ideas to want to do anything anymore. I just want to sit.

Observations

The cognitive observations were that the verbal behaviors continued to reveal no disruptions in the associations. Further, the associations stressed that Mr. M. S. did have a marked alteration in his preinfarct and postinfarct self. Although he depreciated his prior endeavors by labeling them "Johnny-come-lately" and a "complete knowledge of nothing," he clearly had been more vigorous in the past. The affect and physical activity in this segment was more energetic, although once again no dysphoria was manifest. Empathically, one could identify with a man caught up in an emotional paralysis and filled with self-demeaning.

Segment 3

(The patient's last comment was "I just want to sit")

Therapist: You don't have the look or sound of a lazy person. You seem alert and vigorous.

Mr. M. S.: I used to be but I don't have any push. I have no desire anymore. I used to work all day and then come home and decorate and do carpenter work and decorating for other people on Saturday and Sunday to make ends meet. Did all my own automobile servicing where my knowledge was adequate, like changing the oil and putting in new oil filters and things like that. But now, er, everything I want to do, I seem inadequate. I feel like, er, if I'm gonna do anything involving any type of book work, I feel like I've left something out. I feel—what did I miss?

Observations

The observed verbal behavior now reveal Mr. M. S. focusing on two themes: the experience of ineptitude and the absence of motivation. The ineptitude was tied up with the experience of wrongdoing and, further, it reverberated again and again in his thoughts. The affect at the end of the segment became filled with anxiety, and the nonverbal activity became heightened with hand movements accenting his comments. The empathic task in this segment was that of recalling in the therapist's self the ubiquitous experience of feeling inferior and therefore apprehensive in executing a particular assignment felt to be beyond his capacities. The patient made it clear that this self-state of inferiority and fear was not his modal self and therefore represented a transformation of his previous self.

Segment 4

(The last comment was "I feel like I left something out . . . what did I miss?")

Therapist: You question yourself a great deal.
Mr. M. S.: Right. I do. I question myself completely at all times. I
    have no interest in . . . in any festivities. Holiday seasons
    never meant anything to me as far as Christmas or New
    Year's or any of those things. To me, it was a waste of time, a
    waste of effort, to go through all these motions of having a
    good time when you really weren't having a good time. I
    never was interested in buying cards or gifts or anything for
    people. If people were ill, I didn't feel sorry for them like I
    think other people feel sorry for them. You know, no aches or
    pain for their troubles. I figure—well, this is the way it's
    supposed to be, but I steeled myself all through life not to
    show emotion. This has been one of my own doings with
    myself. I never wanted to show emotion of any kind to any-
    body. I wanted to show blank, cold expression.

Observations

The comment "I question myself," etc. indicated Mr. M. S. was vigilant or suspicious or critical towards himself. His next association indicated that he had always been guarded against the emergence of affects of any kind. The restraints that he placed on himself extended into different types of human encounter and involvements from joyous events to illness. His manifest emotions as he related these thoughts showed some sadness, more akin to a somber attitude. In this segment, his body was hunched forward in the chair, and his shoulders and head were less erect.

To empathize with the patient in this segment involved the therapist entering into the world of the outcast, the experience of estrangement from the world of people and whatever they can offer. In some observers this may be a difficult empathic task, to capture in oneself the experience of an outsider, the "underground man" so well described in Dostoyevsky's novella of the same name (Dostoyevsky, 1878/1961). At times, the observer, not having relevant memories to evoke to imagine the self-state of the observed, can utilize personal fantasies assumed to be approximate to the patient, or figures from literature, or other patients. Although these images are not equivalent to one's own remembered self-states, they are helpful in appreciating the patient's inner life. The goal is for the observer to capture the inner self of isolation in order to appreciate the unique experience of the empty, lonely self of the man always on the outside, protecting himself against the human encounters of joy and sadness.

Segment 5

(The patient last said, "I wanted to show blank, cold expression")

Therapist: And sometimes, it seems, maybe even be pleasant or cheerful, hmm?

Mr. M. S.: Cheerful, when I didn't feel cheerful. Yeah.

Therapist: Like today.

Mr. M. S.: Because . . . yes. The situation seemed to call for it so I try to mold my character to what the situation calls for without feeling the, er, feelings that I was supposed to have for the situation. I'm talking to you now but my whole mind isn't given out to you as far as that's concerned. Half my mind is still turned in on me . . . what should I say? or why should I say it? or how am I feeling? But I just don't feel good . . .

Therapist: Mmm-hmm.

Mr. M. S.: . . . mentally. I'm nervous right now and tense. I . . . I take Valiums to reduce my anxiety. I'm a poor sleeper. I take sleeping pills to sleep. I carry nitroglycerin in case I get pains. And sometimes I think my pains are not actual physical pains but brought on by thinking about them, because I've noticed that during the times that I had the angina before I went to the hospital, it always came on when I thought about them or when I did something that I didn't really want to do. When I felt that somebody else should be doing the thing that I'm doing, I'd say, "I'm gonna get a pain" and I'd get a pain. So I, uh . . . when I was in the hospital at the time, I suggested to my doctor that my anginas were caused by emotional problems rather than by actual physical disabilities and I had a Dr. Bushkin come in and see me a couple of times but I couldn't afford psychiatric treatment although I felt I needed it. So he saw me two times in the hospital and said he would see me after he came out—or after I came out—and sent me a bill for $75. I wrote him a letter that I couldn't afford psychiatric fees but I would try a course of self-hypnosis to see if I could relieve my own tensions and feelings, but evidently I wasn't able to. And then not being able to get a job, I went into a business two months ago. I fought going into business for 30 years but not being able to get a job, I went into a business, and the minute I open the door and go in there, I hate the thing like poison. I feel inadequate, inept, unable to run it. The details bother me. It's . . . a bunch of cards come in . . . it's a card and gift store, I get a blank wall, I can't put the cards away. I don't know how to check them in and I think everything has its place and there's a place for everything and when they send in cards that are wrong, I get upset about it. If the price is wrong, I get set up—upset about it. When I order merchandise and only a half order comes in and you've got to check off . . . all this . . . little details bother me terrifically.

Observations

In this segment the patient's restraints weakened and he did relate his current distress: he had been unable to maintain his equilibrium since his heart attack. Currently, he was unable to avoid or suppress his painful experiences of ineptitude in running his business.

The affect now was manifest anxiety in the voice and bodily posture, as well as in the agitated stream of thoughts. The empathic mission in this segment lay in the therapist's need to find in himself a memory of being distraught, being caught up in the psychic disarray of a fragmentation state. A memory of struggling with a difficult mechanical task from childhood would be helpful, or of struggling with an arithmetic problem (long division) or a problem in reading or reading comprehension.

Segment 6

(The patient last said, "Little details bother me terrifically")

Therapist: You mean, [little details] get you angry?

Mr. M. S.: They get me angry plus frustrate me. They frustrate me completely. I-I-I can't explain my full feelings. I can't analyze them. I-I'm just trying to tell you what I feel, but ex-exactly I couldn't say how I feel. But all I feel is useless, that much I know.

Therapist: Even when you talk about the details you find yourself talking with a lot of . . .

Mr. M. S.: Tenseness, yes.

Therapist: . . . irritation.

Mr. M. S.: Irritation. Yes. They bother me. I never did like 'em. . . .

Therapist: Well, let's try to understand that a little better. What is there about these details that gets to you?

Mr. M. S.: Actually, it seems to be the time that it takes to do them—to go from this thing, to this thing, to that thing, back to the other thing. Er, things that only take a minute or two to do in this field to me seem to take eons of time. And not having anything else to do but this thing, I shouldn't feel this way.

Therapist: You have the time.

Mr. M. S.: I have the time. But I feel like I just don't want to do it. I'd rather just sit and look at the wall. I used to read a lot. I don't even have an interest in reading anymore. Practically everything on television bores me. I don't look at it anymore.

Therapist: So you might say that work and the responsibility it entails takes you away from your introversion or withdrawal—takes you away from your thinking blank thoughts.

Mr. M. S.: My self-pity. That's right.

Therapist: Self-pity?

Mr. M. S.: Yes. I–I . . .

Therapist: Is that what you feel when you're looking at a blank wall?

Mr. M. S.: Well, yeah. I look at the blank wall and say, "What the hell, I'm no good for anything anymore," and just sit there and look. I hate to get out of bed in the morning. When I get out of bed in the morning, I-I don't even want to go in to wash or shave, take a shower. I-I . . . a little thing like making the coffee and putting up a slice of toast seems to tire me or just thinking about it tires me. I don't want to do it.

Observations

Mr. M. S. began this segment by describing and revealing his self-state of inadequacy as he mentioned that he could not explain his state of mind nor could he describe with exactness his feeling state. He then went on to describe his increasing withdrawal from the world combined with his difficulty in extricating himself from his hibernation from the world. In this solitude, he could not wash or shave or feed himself because he was so caught up in his withdrawal.

To be able to identify with this self-state of futility is a challenging task for many observers but this is the required frame of reference which the therapist must elicit in his/her memory or imagination. The self-experience of being ill and slowly and painfully recovering at times permits one to vicariously introspect into the patient's experience of futility, fatigue, and the wish for withdrawal from a painful reality. The wretched old man Lear of Shakespeare, railing at his powerlessness, or the aged and raging Oedipus at Colonnus are appropriate images to use if the therapist cannot draw upon adequate sources to empathically understand this segment.

Segment 7

(The patient last said in reference to making coffee and toast, "I don't want to do it")

Therapist: Is there anyone else around to do it?

Mr. M. S.: Not when I get up. My wife is home when, uh, when I get up but she goes to work before I'm ready for breakfast. She would make it if I asked her to but I don't want to be a bother to anybody either in that respect. I've been, more or less, self-sufficient and self-reliant all my life. Did everything myself. Never depended on anybody to do anything. Rather I was doing things for other people at all times. And, er, doing these things, sometimes I felt used or taken advantage of but I did them anyhow and probably stewed about it, er, a little while and then forgot about it but, in times, these things all seemed to build up on me and, er, when I bought this business, against my better judgment—as I saw it—but on impulse, I bought it and without investigating it closely. I talked to people that owned these kind of businesses. They all said, "There's nothing to it." "Simple—just sell cards." They don't tell you about the little old lady that come in and picks up 40 cards and buys one for 15 cents and puts the 40 cards where they are and you gotta go rearrange these 40 cards into their proper categories, their proper pocket, and find the envelopes. And someone with the little kids with their grubby hands that are handling everything that, uh, causes my stomach to curl up and stir in there and I have to take a Valium to relax and. . . .

Observations

The central theme the patient reported in this segment was his disappointment with his human world. He described again his wall against the human encounter and the nurturance he stood against by his lifelong self-sufficiency. However, he then described the paradoxical aspect of his self-reliance and his doing for others: he had commonly felt manipulated by the people in his environment. His next association, thereby connecting it with being used, was to the business he acquired and the tension he had experienced since being in this business. It was in his role as merchant that he now experienced his most intense experience of harassment, since he was being asked again and again to see to others' needs, while his needs for solitude were again not being gratified.

Segment 8

(The patient last stated, "I have to take a Valium to relax")

Therapist: Mmm. Well, this example of people who push you too far . . . what you're saying is that you find yourself taking Valium to cut the level of your anger down.

Mr. M. S.: Anger or anxiety or whatever it may be.

Therapist: What would happen if you didn't cut the level of your irritation down?

Mr. M. S.: Oh, my stomach would tie into a knot. I'd get tense right in here. I'd be . . . and then I'd think bad thoughts and I might go off thinking about . . . what the hell's the use of hanging around here . . . see . . . kill myself or something like that. This is . . . this is. . . .

Therapist: Kill yourself?

Mr. M. S.: Kill myself.

Therapist: You never think about discharging your irritation at the person who angered you?

Mr. M. S.: Never. Never thought about anybody else except that *I* feel myself inadequate, inept, and that I think I'm not any use to anybody anymore and the easiest way to get rid of all my problems would be to end it all. That's the thoughts that I've had. I have this business. I have it only two months and I hate it. I want to sell it. I want to get out of it but you cannot sell a business overnight so I have to go down there every day and stew with it and buy merchandise. I don't even think . . . I can't even figure out who to call to buy or ask to get the merchandise. I–I draw a perfect blank when it comes to that. I've never been in business. Everybody tells me, do this and do that, and as soon as they tell me, I forget to do it or who to call or what to do and then I think about . . . well, a lady comes in and asks for two of these things and I call up a place . . . I finally get a number of . . . and they say, "You can't buy two, you've got to buy a dozen." So I say to myself, "Well, gee, if I'm only gonna sell two, I've gotta buy a dozen and there's 10 or so to stand around the shelf. This is merchandise money I've got put in there. I don't know if I'm ever gonna sell them or not." I don't know what to buy or how to buy it because I've never been in this kind of business before or any kind of business where I had to be the bookkeeper, merchandiser, the salesman, the buyer, the . . . well, what is there to running a business? You have to be about 19 different people in a small, little, one-man shop like I have, and I feel inadequate to do all these things.

Observations

The observations of the verbal behavior now showed Mr. M. S.'s continuing preoccupation with the two themes: his inferiority in tandem with a milieu of customers and relatives who were not responding to his weaknesses of mind and body. In the beginning of this segment, the patient *connected* his deep sense of futility and inadequacy with an admixture of suicidal thoughts and the experience on his part that he was no longer an active producer, an achieving man. He continued to reveal this pervasive mood of resignation from the world. The affect and other nonverbal behaviors in this segment contained the affect and behavior of agitation, a man caught up in the experience of yet *another* attack on him by the uncontrollable forces of his environment.

Empathically speaking, the therapist must search deeply to capture a memory of a self-scenario that is a good "fit" with the patient's. In this segment Mr. M. S. was informing the therapist of the reactivity he had experienced in relation to "slight" (i.e., insults), the reaction of an unempathic environment.

Segment 9

(The patient last stated, "I feel inadequate to do all these things")

Mr. M. S.: The family has offered to help and do the things for me but I don't want to be a burden on them. I don't want to cause them to have to do these things for me. Like I say, I've been. . . .

Therapist: Mmm-hmm.

Mr. M. S.: I feel absolutely inadequate for it. They are helping me to the extent that they can but they want me to do the things for myself also so that I will learn what I have to do. But I don't want to and this is the problem. I don't want to learn.

Therapist: Mmm-hmm. But you started the shop on your own volition? It was your idea?

Mr. M. S.: It was a seed planted in my mind by one of the relatives. Of my own volition, I never would have thought or . . . of going into business. I never desired to go into business. It was a seed that was planted and it grew and grew and grew and I just did it on impulse, like that, a hunch, whatever you want to call it. And I should never do things like that 'cause I've been unlucky all my life as far as hunches and impulses were concerned. This is another phobia that I have—that I'm extremely unlucky in my complete life, although I have a lovely wife, three children, and two lovely grandchildren. But, er, that's the way I feel.

Therapist: Now which relative was it that planted this idea?

Mr. M. S.: My son-in-law. He has a newspaper agency. He would . . . he would love to have the store for himself right now but the business he has takes 20 hours a day of his time and he cannot put another 20 hours in at another job. It was the desire of his all the time to get into a field like this. He says he'd love it. I says, "Take it (*laughs*), I'll give it to you. I can't stand it." He says, "I can't. I've got this other business. I can't do anything with it." So it was an impulse and it was a bad impulse—taking whatever I had, as far as cash is concerned, and this is also a worry with me. I want to get out of it and—as fast as I can—lose as little as possible because I feel it's a thing that I cannot handle.

Observations

In this segment, the main themes continued to be those of a man immersed in the experience of massive inferiority. Mr. M. S. continued to rail at himself: he is a burden, he cannot succeed in business, he is a man marked with poor luck, he has been too impulsive. In his current self-state, he demeaned his painful experiences as "laziness" or "stubbornness."

The nonverbal behavior revealed some expression of anger in discussing his son-in-law's refusal to take over the business. An observer ordinarily cannot match through empathic means of appreciation the pervasive ineptitude and self-demeaning of this patient, which in itself is an important diagnostic observation, but one can arrive at an approximation of this person's self-state which will be sufficient to appreciate the despair of his self.

Segment 10

(The patient in speaking of his business, has said, "I want to get out of it")

Therapist: Mmm-hmm. Well, what were your hopes of it?

Mr. M. S.: Of what?

Therapist: The business. Why did you find yourself going into business? What did you want?

Mr. M. S.: I wanted to be useful and to work and, uh, try to make a living but I found that this is not for me. There are some people that are business men and some people that are working men. I'm a working man. Been a working man all my life—a producer—worked in a cleaning plant for 30 years without any technical knowledge of the cleaning industry, but I worked myself up from a little—what you call a flunky— to silk spotter in 30 years and the last 20 years of it, I was the head silk spotter. Worked myself up in 10 years to that and I was adequate. I did the job very good. Even doing that and knowing that I was doing a good job, there are some people that are chronic complainers that if you do a thing as perfect or as well as it can be done, they'll always say it was not good for some reason or other. There are people like that and this used to bother me, too, even in a field that I knew I was doing as well as could be expected. When somebody would make a fuss, I felt inadequate then, too.

Therapist: So you've always had a tendency to doubt yourself.

Mr. M. S.: An infer . . . doubt myself, yes.

Therapist: Mmm-hmm.

Mr. M. S.: Although I put on a big front not to let people know this. I concealed it. I always put on a big ego, you know—a big know-it-all, eh, and an anticonformist, if you want to call it that. If people always wear ties, I don't like ties. I don't wear ties. If people all rush downtown because the president came in to—to go down State Street, I says, "He's just another man, I'm not interested in going down to see another man." Everybody, years ago, everybody used to wear wide brim hats. I didn't think I looked good in a wide brim hat; I wore a narrow brim hat. I didn't believe in style. Now everybody's wearing continental clothes, I still wear pleats because I feel more comfortable in pleats. They . . . they all call me a rugged individualist. Well, this is probably a front that I was putting up but I . . . I never followed the crowd. I wasn't what . . . like I used to call people sheep. There's one with the bell. He leads the way and everybody follows. I've never had the desire to follow—to be a follower. Yet, I don't have the education or the know-how to be a leader. So I pretended, more or less, to, uh, know or talk about things that were current, at the moment, to be a leader.

Therapist: What do you mean, pretended?

Mr. M. S.: Well, I talk with . . . with force . . . or with emphasis and, er, quote figures or cite figures that I read or thought I read and . . . but . . . like I knew what I was talking about.

Therapist: What do you think you're doing now in telling me about these qualities?

Mr. M. S.: What . . . I'm just talking to you. That's all I'm doing. I'm trying . . . I'm trying to tell my character and my feelings to you so that you can tell me what's wrong with me and give me the . . . what I need to get over the feelings that I feel.

Therapist: Aren't you kind of knocking yourself though?

Mr. M. S.: I'm always knocking myself.

Therapist: This is what's been going on with you, the last . . .

Mr. M. S.: Oh, yeah. Oh, yes.

Therapist: . . . several months.

Mr. M. S.: Oh, yes. Always knocking myself.

Therapist: Ever since . . .

Mr. M. S.: Belittling myself.

Therapist: . . . ever since the coronary.

Mr. M. S.: That's right.

Therapist: Not before that, you said.

Mr. M. S.: Not . . . not, er, generally, only occasionally.

Therapist: Yeah. But these days, this is what you do.

Mr. M. S.: That's right. Continuously.

Observations

The verbal behavior in this last segment now revealed a man who was speaking more freely, with more vigor, and was now not as retarded in associations or in affect. As previously, the content of Mr. M. S.'s comments in this segment dealt with the weakened self, burdened with doubts and recriminations, a man ever eager to label himself a fraud. This segment revealed two new observations: 1) the comment that he had experienced the feeling of inadequacy in the past when rebuffed; 2) the comment that he wished to overcome his feelings with the help of the therapist.

The observer should be able to undergo an empathic shift with this new material—verbal and nonverbal—which now evokes empathic resonances that are less dire than when Mr. M. S. started the interview announcing that he felt suicidal. Now the observer's empathy may turn, for example, to remembrances of himself hanging back from an intimidating social setting and compensating for the experienced inferiority by uttering disparaging remarks at the event and the people involved.

SUMMARY

We have been emphasizing that the credo of the psychotherapist is "Data, more data." Another emphasis proceeding from this one is that our communications of our observations to each other and to our patients state our *findings*, not our "sense of" or "my fantasy" type of comments. We have by now sufficiently stressed the two major types of observations—cognitive and empathic— and their respective data-gathering methodologies. It should perhaps be reemphasized that these two sets of observations enable the observer to be in touch with his patient's involvement in his interpersonal world (cognitive observations) and his intrapsychic world (empathic observations). These two sets of observations have their own special value; the observer of the interview must be diligent in securing both these data bases for the complete appraisal of the patient.

We have thus far omitted the effect on the patient of the ambience created in this unusual setting where all attention is on the patient's issues. This atmosphere of caring is for many patients an unusual happening: in almost all interviews or therapeutic sessions the communication mode established between interviewer or therapist and patient is a monologue and never a genuine dialogue. This total attention from the therapist is experienced by many patients as uplifting or invigorating. For others, this spotlighting experience evokes their *defenses* against unfolding themselves to anticipated rejection, resulting in the long periods of withdrawal in interviews until—hopefully—they achieve the experience of being in a safe environment. The considerations listed above enable the interviewer to be ever mindful of the impact of the interview process on a variety of people: some require of their therapists restraint in manner; others may require more interaction; but all require a tailor-made posture on the part of the therapist to ensure their cohesiveness as they unfold their difficulties in the diagnostic phase.

We have not yet spoken of the impact on the interviewer of becoming a professional or inveterate observer of others. Becoming a trenchant observer of verbal and nonverbal behavior in one's human milieu does offer a keener appreciation of the environment. But it is important to be aware of the occupational hazard of always being an observer; one must remember to interact, at least now and then! The same considerations apply to being aware of the hazards of being a constant empathizer with others so that each interpersonal involvement is directed to the other person's gain to the exclusion of one's own goals. A more significant positive transformation of the therapist's self takes place as a result of a focus on becoming a professional or inveterate observer of the human encounter. Apart from the occupational hazards mentioned, the professional empathic and cognitive observer does have a keener involvement in all that he/she surveys with these new lenses. Becoming a consistent empathizer and introspecter enriches life and indeed does instill a sense of joy, although most often a joy that is subdued since the contents of what one is in touch with in another person are often not joyous. The sense of joy refers to the ever-increasing ability to identify, albeit transiently, with the psychological condition of the other. This sense of joy is experienced when one can capture the self-state of a figure from a novel or play as well as in an interview setting. All of a sudden the therapist becomes aware that one's listening is never casual; it always involves following associations, observing affect, and attempting to appreciate the other's inner experience, whether the other is a patient, a colleague, or a figure in a novel.

It is, in our view, a gratifying self-transformation.

The next chapter gives an introduction to the findings and theories of self psychology, especially stressing the development of the self and the model of self-pathology. This chapter is of special significance in understanding the definitive chapters that follow on the psychotherapeutic modalities.

2

The Development of
the Self and the
Model of Self-Pathology

In Kohut's view, the self is considered the center of the psychological universe (Kohut, 1977), by which he meant that man can
only be understood in terms of his experiences—his inner mental
life—not his behavior (Kohut, 1959). It follows from this that any
genuine investigation of man must be through the medium of
empathy—vicarious introspection—which therefore defines and
restricts the observational field of psychological understanding.

Thus, the self is the center of the personality. As Kohut (1977)
stated:

> The self is the core of our personality. It has various constitu-
> ents which we acquire in the interplay with those persons in
> our earliest childhood environment whom we experience as
> selfobjects. A firm self, resulting from optimal interactions
> between the child and his selfobjects, is made up of the three
> major constituents: 1) one pole from which emanates the
> basic strivings for power and success; 2) another pole that
> harbors the basic idealized goals; and 3) an intermediate area

26

of basic talents and skills that are activated by the tension arc that establishes itself between ambitions and ideals. (p. 180)

According to Kohut (1977), the complete self is a supraordinate structure which functions not only as the receiver of impressions derived from the environment but as the center of action and is experienced as continuous in space and time—a cohesive entity. As noted above, the self can be further identified in terms of its major constituents, the so-called bipolar self. These poles of the self come into their final form through interaction with the significant persons in infancy and childhood who function as the instigators of these self-functions. The pole of ambitions comes into being as a result of special activities of the parent who functions as an admirer–approver–echoer of the unfolding self and thus offers to the child an experience of unquestioning confirmation of the child's worth. From the view of the child, this parent is experienced as a separate entity, over which, however, he or she has total control—much as one controls various parts of one's body. Hence the designation *selfobject*, in this case, the mirroring selfobject.

These early relationships are experienced as fusions or mergers, i.e., immersions (psychologically speaking) into the body and mind of the caretaking selfobject. Establishing the archaic self/selfobject mirroring dyad is crucial for psychological life. However, for structure building to take place, the self-aggrandizing mirror functions must be *interiorized* or *internalized*, i.e., become an actual addition to the contents of the self so that self-esteem—an intrapsychic function—replaces selfobject mirroring—an interpersonal activity (Val, 1982). In Kohut's view, internalization of selfobject mirroring functions takes place along the lines first articulated by Freud in "Mourning and Melancholia," which described the mourner's unique reaction to loss—internalization of significant aspects of the departed person—as a ubiquitous reaction to separation (Freud, 1917a).

At about the same time in an infant's development the second major influence on self-development occurs. It is the establishment of the idealizing parental imago selfobject. Where the mirroring selfobjects are those who respond to and confirm the infant's grandiosity, the idealized parent imago are figures whom the child looks up to and merges with as an imago of calmness, soothing, and perfection, and thus a source of strength. One other early self/selfobject experience is ordinarily present in the child's ontogeny, namely, the experience of what Kohut (1977) called the alter-ego–twinship merger in which the child experiences the parent self essentially the same as his or her own self. This essential sameness is instrumental in enhancing the child's skills and unfolding his or her talents, as well as forming the anlage for the later-life experience and need for togetherness and alliance (Kohut, 1977).

The next phase of the child's development is significant in the formation of the cohesive self; it is the step of internalization of the selfobject's functions of initiating and promoting esteem so that what was a feature of the self/selfobject relationship now becomes a set of self-functions. Kohut (1971) described the interiorization of these functions as occurring in two steps: 1) optimal frustrations and 2) transmuting internalization.

Optimal frustrations refer to the unavoidable disappointments in child rearing such that the child does not obtain the instant feedback that he or she may be demanding. These unavoidable delays, absences, misappreciations, which are not protracted or in any way traumatic (optimal frustrations), promote the internalization of the mirroring or other selfobject functions so that the child now has the mirroring selfobject's approval attached, so to speak, to his or her self as a permanent source of nurturance (transmuting internalization) (Kohut, 1971). Over time the sequence of optimal frustrations leading to transmuting internalization proceeds to a cohesive self, so that one can identify a nuclear self. This structure is bipolar in its psychological shape, one pole representing the transformed archaic grandiosity in the pole of ambitions, the other pole representing the internalized archaic idealizations in the transformed pole of ideals. This early self, which can now be labeled the nuclear self, thus has a pole of ambitions which strives to live up to its pole of ideals through the talents and skills of the self (Tolpin, 1971). In fact, in the adult self, the cohesion of the self is maintained through the tension arc created by the pole of ambitions striving to live up to the ideals through the exertions of the talents and skills in what Kohut called a program of action:

> With the term tension arc, however, I am referring to the abiding flow of actual psychological activity that establishes itself between the two poles of the self; i.e., a person's basic pursuits towards which he is driven by his ambitions and led by his ideals. (Kohut, 1977, p. 180)

The bipolar self now experienced by the child as continuous in time and discrete in space maintains its cohesiveness—its resistance to breakup (fragmentation)—through two sources of self-cement. One is the pool of endogenous stores of self-support derived from the internalized functions of selfobjects maintaining self-esteem; the other is the continuing need for selfobjects throughout life. Kohut's (1977) finding was that self/selfobject relationships formed the essence of psychological life from birth to death.

Kohut described, as noted, the essence of psychological life in terms of the nature of the self/selfobject relationship, which, however, changes over time and in functioning. The earliest self/selfobject contacts, as previously noted, are actually merging types of relationships; they actually instill esteem in the child, after optimal frustration.

From the archaic selfobject relationships there is a developmental line of self/selfobject encounters to what is called the mature selfobject relationships which offer an experience of empathic resonance—the admiration of a colleague through which the adult self can experience a revival of the memory traces of the archaic selfobject's mirroring or calming and soothing, and in this manner restore a disequilibrium due to a temporary flagging of esteem. Throughout one's development the self requires selfobject refueling to maintain the integrity of the self. At times these selfobject encounters will approach the approving–admiring–calming–

merging interactions resembling the archaic self/selfobject fusions.

Thus, in the anal stage of development, the child's need for the mirroring responses of the selfobject parent are necessary so that the child's toilet-training accomplishments are given value. In the oedipal phase of development, the child's selfobject requirement of his or her parents is that they respond to his or her increased assertiveness in sexual and other spheres with admiration and pride at the vigor and creativeness displayed. In these early stages of development it seems clear that the selfobject encounters, while not of the early archaic types, still continue to provide supportive experiences which will be internalized and serve to enhance the achievements of the youngster in his or her development.

In adolescence the need for the mirroring selfobject parent to give credence to the creative activities is time-honored. It is also well-known how intense is the need in the adolescent for an intimate contact with an idealized selfobject. In both of these instances, again internalization of selfobject functioning is effected.

In later life, as Kohut (1977) stated, self/selfobject encounters continue to provide necessary refueling of one's worth through mature selfobject encounters and the phenomenon of empathic resonance. In old age, for example, the need for mirroring of one's achievements and of one's courage in the face of death is necessary (Kohut, 1971).

In sum, the self is maintained in a cohesive manner through the strength of its constituents, the firm sense of assertiveness, the intact sense of one's values serving as a compass through life, and the ability to exert one's skills and talents in the pursuit of one's programs of action from writing a speech to caring for the disabled. Selves differ considerably in the relative weaknesses or strengths of their constituents. Overall, there are selves that are firm or enfeebled, resistant to fragmentation (cohesive) or highly vulnerable to losses of worth and thus prone to fragmentation. There are selves that are intensely firm in the pole of assertiveness, the charismatic selves, and there are selves that are highly leadership-oriented, the messianic selves. Some selves are mirror-hungry, while others are chronically searching for a leader (Kohut & Wolf, 1978).

PATHOLOGY OF SELF OR SELF-DISORDERS

The position of self psychology is that all forms of psychopathology are ultimately derived from defects in the overall structure of the self or from distortions of the self, both of them due to disturbances of self/selfobject relationships in childhood. (Further, self psychology asserts that, in contrast to classical analysis, the conflicts in the object–instinctual realm—i.e., in the realm of object love and object hate, in particular the set of conflicts called the oedipus complex—are not the cause of psychopathology, but its results [Kohut, 1977].)

As we previously have seen, the self, in adult life as well as in childhood, will be in a state of cohesiveness, harmony, or fragmentation, i.e., it will be enfeebled, distorted, or firm—all resulting from the success or failure of the archaic self/selfobject relationships. Should there be a failure in the self/selfobject relationships in childhood or adult life, certain consequences will obtain. One such consequence is the painful experience of a massive failure of the self/selfobject relationships, the experience of fragmentation. Fragmentation in the view of self psychology is the central pathological experience referring to the self breakdown and is ushered in by a massive loss of self-esteem, followed immediately by the advent of the global anxiety referred to as disintegration anxiety. Directly after the advent of disintegration anxiety, the self is experienced as losing its cohesiveness with the usual experience of splitting or fragmentation of the self-functions and self-perceptions, including the self-functions of reality testing, memory, orientation of space and time, and the loss of the intact experience of self-observing. The various experiences of the different organs, previously coalesced together in the intact experience of the total bodyself, are now experienced as separate and become foci for enhanced attention and even preoccupation to the point of hypochondria. Finally, a failure in a self/selfobject encounter will commonly lead to a rage reaction that is unique. These eruptions of rage, the so-called narcissistic rage reactions, are without a purpose, save to vent destructiveness on anyone in their immediate environment. It is one of the ubiquitous responses to the experience of losing control over one's selfobjects (Kohut, 1971).

A self/selfobject failure in childhood has different consequences from a self/selfobject failure in adult life. In adult life, the cohesive self has continuing selfobject encounters which are of value in maintaining the cohesiveness of the self; i.e., mature selfobject encounters result in continuing support to the self through empathic resonance, by supplying mirroring or firmness to add to the cohesiveness of the self. A failed selfobject encounter in adulthood will ordinarily, in a cohesive self, lead to a transitory fragmentation with hypochondria, loss of esteem, temporary interference in mentation, and so forth.

However, a massive failure or chronic failure during the phases of childhood when the self is unfolding may result in a fragmentation that will eventually be resolved, i.e., the self will reconstitute itself (the fragmentation will subside), but the self will now have permanent alterations. The overall experience of the self will be that of a self chronically low in energy, i.e., a self depleted of vigor and without evidence of the experience of joy. This self will be quite reactive to criticism and failures by becoming more withdrawn or at times caught up in the explosion of a narcissistic rage reaction which, as stated previously, represents the reaction to the loss of control of the functions of the selfobject and, therefore, is without an object for ventilation of the rage. Depending on the specific type of selfobject failures, the resulting self-distortion may be that of a self weakened in its poles of assertiveness or ideals, or in the areas of its talents and skills. These defects will of course lead to the absence of formulated programs of action in life (in educational, athletic, or musical pursuits, for example).

The overall result of such self/selfobject failures may be a self that experiences life as being empty and that is constantly in the throes of loneliness. This self may be quite resistant to human encounters and, although it experiences loneliness and has desires for human encounters, maintains a conscious attitude of haughtiness and isolation. At times this self may attempt to gain self-esteem support through a variety of activities designed to enhance the chronic emptiness, such as compulsive homo- or heterosexuality, bouts of addiction to substances to provide calming experiences, or compulsive episodes of stealing to enhance esteem. At other times the selfobject failures in childhood eventuate in what appears to be a syndrome of neurosis.

These reactions occur when after a failed selfobject encounter, such as a failure of mirroring in the oedipal phase of childhood, the child becomes preoccupied with the particular phase-specific drive or phase-specific developmental task which ultimately leads to a *fixation* on the particular drive or developmental task. The failure of a self/selfobject encounter during the oedipal phase of development leads to a child permanently preoccupied with the fears of that phase in life which were never allayed (Basch, 1981; Muslin, 1985; Tolpin, 1978; Wolf, 1980). Thus an oedipal fixation or an anal fixation represents a failed self/selfobject relationship of that developmental era of childhood.

The secondary elaborations of the self breakdown at those specific times in childhood when developmental tasks needed to be mastered, with the usual addition of the selfobject functions of mirroring or guidance, are in the nature of the exaggerated attention on the drive currently in focus and the defenses elaborated in an attempt to ameliorate or repress the exaggerated drive fragments.

To repeat, the sequence of the self-dissolution into the psychopathological forms previously outlined is as follows: The cohesive self, in response to a self/selfobject rupture, breaks down or becomes fragmented, which then may take one of several pathways. The fragmented self may maintain a state of *chronic fragmentation* (protracted fragmentation disorders, borderline personalities); the fragmented self may repair itself without evidence of the previous state of breakdown (episodic fragmentation); the fragmented self will reequilibrate itself with newly developed defenses against selfobject bonds (narcissistic personality disorders); the fragmented self will focus on the drives which are in focus as part of the current developmental phase or activated as a manifestation of a regressive reaction (neurotic syndromes) and secondarily develop defenses against the egress of the specifically elaborated drives (Kohut, 1971, 1977).

Episodic Fragmentation Disorders

Reactions to a breakdown in self/selfobject bonds are of course ubiquitous, since self/selfobject bonds and failures are ubiquitous. As have been described, selfobject involvements range from those archaic self/selfobject ties that continue over time to those selfobjects that are experienced as so-called mature selfobject encounters. In adults, the need to enter into an archaic self/selfobject bond is limited to those instances in which the self is subjected to psychological trauma requiring a temporary merging relationship. These are, of course, instances in which the self is suddenly devoid of narcissistic supplies and is in need of the experience of fusion with a mirroring selfobject or a revered leader. Archaic self/selfobject bonds are always in the service of investing the self with the experience of worth, of strength, of calming and soothing. In childhood, these experiences give the self the requisite strength of cohesion; in adulthood they effect a repair to a fragmenting self when entered into temporarily in relation to the stress of dissolution. Mature selfobject encounters are those interactions in which the self is in need of a temporary enhancement of esteem, i.e., a self-situation of esteem-deficiency such as is experienced in the innumerable states of self-doubt. Here the self-experiences of the selfobject are in actuality not those of an object fused with one's self and under one's control, but rather the self has a reactivation of the early self/selfobject mergers and experiences a state of esteem enhancement, thus effecting a repair of the self's cohesion. Seen in this way, much of adult interactional life consists of mature selfobject encounters with others who function temporarily to repair a flagging self-esteem or with symbolic encounters with music or literature in which the self is uplifted or invigorated.

Thus, episodic fragmentations or near-fragmentations or simple instances of loss of esteem or threatened loss of worth are part of one's modal reactions to a complex world of victories, near-misses, and failures. In a more-or-less cohesive self, the repair in most instances will be effected by entering into a so-called mature self/selfobject encounter. In those instances where the demands for cohesion are intense, the previously cohesive self will fragment, albeit temporarily, and seek out an archaic self/selfobject encounter in which a merger will be effected. For example, the psychological reactions of the person who has just been informed that her long-standing state of weakness is due to a malignancy in her colon frequently are the self-experience of fragmentation. Hopefully the individual's distress will be followed by the self/selfobject merger effected with a trusted caretaker or relative. In these situations, the fragmentation experience is short-lived if empathic caretakers recognize the manifestations of the fragmentation and respond appropriately with a dose of mirroring or by allowing themselves to become the target for idealization (Kohut & Wolf, 1978).

Self-Fragmentation Resulting in Neurotic Syndromes

In the view of self psychology, drives come into focus when the self is fragmenting, hence the designation that drives are disintegration products of a fragmenting self (Kohut, 1977). From this vantage point, consider the self of the oedipal phase child and his/her selfobject needs for his emerging phase-specific assertiveness, including his sexual assertiveness of a homoerotic and heteroerotic nature (in each case with hostility towards the opposite parent). If the situation obtains that the selfobject supports are missing or inadequate and the child experiences the parents' withdrawal or rejection of him during this important phase in his development, the self-depletion will result in a fragmented self. The result will, in some instances, be not an eruption of the so-called narcissistic rage but a preoccupation with the drives derailed from the now-fragmented self. In the ordinary functions of the self, the drives are a vital part of the self-seeking and maintaining contact with the world, including the world of selfobjects. In a fragmented self, the drives are now in a free state and clearly visible since they are not bound up with the functions of the cohesive self.

Returning to the oedipal child whose self, now in a fragmented condition, will have unleashed "oedipal" drives, these phase-specific drives will eventuate in repetitive experiences of anxiety, centering on tissue destruction—the so-called castration anxiety with its attendant features of anxiety dreams of mutilation—and the buildup of irrational guilt. Self psychology argues, in disagreement with classical psychoanalysis, that the emergence of the oedipal neurosis or oedipal complex is a result of the failure of the selfobjects of the oedipal phase whose failures usher in, first the fragmentation of the self followed by the child's repetitious preoccupation with the assertions specific to the oedipal phase and the subsequent fears and guilts. Self psychology further holds that if a child in the oedipal phase of development becomes the recipient of helpful selfobject supports, he or she will emerge from this normal phase of development, the oedipal phase, with heteroerotic and homoerotic strivings with a minimum of guilt and castration. In contradistinction to classical psychoanalysis, self psychology does not regard the oedipal phase as "the pivotal point regarding the fate of the self that it is with regard to the formation of the psychic apparatus" (Kohut, 1977, p. 240).

In sum, the neurotic syndromes, which in classical psychoanalysis emerge from the predetermined unfolding of the drives coming into intense conflict with ego defenses and superego, are conceptualized in self psychology as one of the possible outcomes of a self in fragmentation. Self psychology holds that if the self is intact, no preoccupation with the drives in an isolated fashion takes place. Thus from the viewpoint of the self psychologist, although an oedipal phase of development is a ubiquitous happening, if there is an adequate set of selfobjects the child emerges with a firming up of assertiveness that is now more adequately controlled with a firming up of the gender experience. Contrariwise, if there has been a selfobject failure to the modal egress of assertiveness in an oedipal youngster, the derailed (unattached) instinctual drives will be seen as naked lust and hostility.

The Narcissistic Personality and Behavior Disorders

Self/selfobject failures during the phase of the early development of the self, when protracted, result in a variety of self-disorders. Those self disorders, called the narcissistic personality disorders, and the acting-out variety of this disorder, the narcissistic behavior disorders, ordinarily result from a failure of functioning of the mirroring selfobject and an inability of the idealized parent to compensate for the primary selfobject failure (Kohut, 1977). The resultant self is one in which the cohesiveness of the total self is defective and both poles of the self are inadequately filled. This self is vulnerable to fragmentation, especially in relation to further losses of esteem from its milieu. The self-experience is commonly a reflection of the diminutive poles of assertiveness and ideals; thus, the common experience is one of emptiness and/or loneliness. However, the self-needs for mirroring or leadership are commonly defended against by attitudes of haughtiness and superciliousness, reflecting the anxiety towards allowing any further selfobject encounters to transpire. Another common experience in persons with these disorders is to become immersed in transitory relationships in which an archaic self/selfobject dyad is formed and then rejected ordinarily out of a mixture of anticipated psychic pain and disappointment since the relationship cannot offer them the longed-for childhood gratification. Fragmentation states commonly lead to intense loss of esteem, the so-called empty depression, i.e., without prominent guilt. Other common features of the fragmentation states are the experience of disintegration anxiety—an anxiety state marked by panicky feelings, dissociations, end-of-the-world sensations—followed by mentational dysfunctioning (memory loss, reality-testing deficits, loss of synthesizing, and the appearance of derailing of associations) and hypochondriasis. The hypochondriasis in fragmentation states reflect the state of the "unglued" self.

While the ordinary experience of a single organ or anatomical part is minimal in a cohesive self, when the self is fragmenting, a particular organ percept in the self now functionally split off from the rest of the self may be suddenly experienced in a highly charged fashion. A patient in the middle of a fragmentation reaction may complain of unusual body feelings and localize them to an awareness that her face or nose or abdomen is now experienced quite differently: it seems too large, too prominent. These experiences reflect the body percepts becoming split off, and for the first time, prominent in the patient's awareness. The patients with narcissistic personality disorders at times exhibit behavior which expresses their reactions to insult or their needs for calming and soothing or mirroring. These narcissistic behavior disorders encompass the behavior of the compulsive homosexual, the addict, and those delinquents who steal as a symbolic expression of the self need for a selfobject gift. Those addicts who experience the compound and the effects of the compound as an aid to calming and soothing are clearly demonstrating and gratifying archaic self-needs, as well as those homosexuals who feel mirrored in frantically sought-out episodes of fellatio. The patients who suffer with narcissistic personality disorders do not experience protracted fragmentation states; their fragmentation is transitory, and ordinarily these patients seek relief, complaining of their experience of isolation and their inability to form and maintain human relationships.

In sum, those patients with these self-disorders have had failures in their self/selfobject relationships early in life. In effect they have fixation of their self-developments and thus continue—albeit unconsciously—to effect repeated archaic self/selfobject bonds to no avail since they will shortly reject these relationships. The failure of adequate internalizations of the selves of these patients leads to the vulnerability to fragmentation states, which in these patients is resolved by the self-capacity to erect firm defenses against the egress of the self-desires for empathic understanding and gratification.

Protracted Fragmentation States

Patients with borderline disorders and psychoses of all kinds demonstrate not only a heightened vulnerability to self-fragmentation but also a protracted quality to their fragmentation. When a borderline patient develops a fragmentation state which is followed by reality-testing loss (psychosis), derailing, and other symptoms of an acute psychotic decompensation, these pathological states may persist for a long time. Further, these patients do not have an adequate capacity to form a therapeutic self/selfobject dyad based on an alliance of effort to appreciate their inner mental life. These patients commonly experience an absence of as-if transference phenomena and develop a transference psychosis, insisting that the therapist feels this or that and now wishes to cause the patient harm. Thus, in all instances of these patients who have protracted fragmentations, the history reveals that the patient was and is the victim of grossly inadequate selfobject dyads. The result of these failures was the absence of internalization of selfobject functioning (such as admiring), and thus the selves of these people are permanently liable to fragmentations.

SUMMARY

To conclude this chapter, one could say that the central teaching of Kohut in the area of psychopathological syndromes is that all forms of psychopathology are due to disturbances of self/selfobject relationships which result in structural defects in the self and render that self vulnerable to fragmentation and the vicissitudes of fragmentation. Whereas Freud's model of the mind posits that erupting instinctual derivatives come into conflict with the superego and ego—the model of the structural theory—and lead to new defenses (neurotic symptoms), the Kohutian model teaches that one must empathize with the self which is fragmenting due to a current self-deficit of cohesiveness brought about by loss of esteem from whatever source. The Kohutian model focuses on the self-in-fragmentation as the initial manifestation of psychic disequilibrium which may lead to an episodic fragmentation, a chronic fragmentation, the syndrome of repression of self-needs defended by self-attitudes of haughtiness and superciliousness, or the neurosis which represents the psyche focused on the drives that are disintegration products of the fragmenting self.

3

The Empathic Diagnosis and the Therapeutic Diagnosis

Perhaps the most important task in performing psychotherapy is the diagnosis of the self-deficits and of the areas of the self that are intact, here referred to as the empathic diagnosis. Another essential task is that of matching the difficulties and the strengths of the self of the patient with the appropriate therapy, the therapeutic diagnosis. This chapter will serve as a model for the mode of teaching that we will be pursuing throughout this volume, a model of teaching that centers on learner and teacher sharing the observed data.

THE EMPATHIC DIAGNOSIS

An empathic diagnosis begins with the intent on the interviewer's part to identify—albeit transiently—with the self of the subject he is observing in order to appreciate the other's experience. The empathic diagnosis is an assessment of the subject's experiences of himself which the observer will ultimately gather together to form a model of the observed self. The diagnosis is founded on accurate cognitive observations of the manifest verbal behavior— the verbal associations judged as to fit, tempo, and logicality—and the nonverbal behaviors including affects—their appropriateness, mobility, and modulation of the affects—and the other nonverbal behaviors such as gait, grooming, and gestures. Above all, the empathic diagnosis rests on the observer's self-observing capacity to approximate the self of the patient. Whether this is accomplished through vicarious introspection, i.e., through the observer drawing on a memory of a self-state that is surmised to be congruent with the patient's self, or through remembrances of other patients' psychological experiences, or simply through imagining the patient's self-state by referring to memories of literary characters, the operational task is to view the world from the eyes of the patient (Kohut, 1959).

The empathic attitude towards data gathering implies that the observer is optimally free from bias or other resistances to empathy so that a minimum of distortion of the observed data takes place. There are, however, interferences with empathic observations and these interferences take two forms: one is the resistance to the use of empathy; the other lies in the area of empathic inaccuracies. In the case of the resistance to the use of empathy, the observer's empathic shutdown is commonly based on disavowal—the unconscious repudiation of the meaning of the patient's material which has evoked distressful reactions in the observer. In this situation, the observer's capacity to sit in the patient's shoes has become blocked and he, the observer, is interacting with the patient as one civilian to another, rather than as an observer empathizing with a patient's unique self-state (Muslin, 1974, 1984; Muslin & Schlessinger, 1971).

The second problem area in empathic observation—that of empathic inaccuracies—has many roots. In some instances of empathic inaccuracy the observer's pool of self-state memories that are congruent with the self of the patient is absent and he, the observer, is limited in all other avenues of imagination to discern the self he is observing. In other instances, the observer inadvertently has had a transference reaction to the patient and thus will be bound by his experience of his transference onto the patient rather than immersing himself in the patient's self-state (Wolf, 1983).

The next stage in the empathic diagnosis of our subject is to organize the empathically derived data into a model of the mind that ultimately enables us to prescribe a relevant mode of therapy for this particular self (Gedo & Goldberg, 1973). The model of the mind that the therapist uses, whether it be the drive-defense model of classical psychoanalysis or the model of psychoanalytic self psychology, must address itself to the following consider-ations: What is amiss or deficient in the self from the subject's view of himself or from the reaction of his environment that may be critical and rejecting of him? What is deficient in the patient's functioning, from the point of view of the observer, be it his capac-ity for action or his capacity to maintain and pursue goals or standards for himself, or his incapacity to extricate himself from the walls he has built against making contact with people?

The self-model of the mind, which was described in the pre-vious chapter, posits a bipolar self (Kohut, 1977). One pole is the pole of ambitions which is an attempt to describe one set of func-tions of the cohesive self, those functions involved in mastering the environment that include securing approval from one's friend or mate. This pole ordinarily develops through the vicissitudes of sufficient admiring and approving from a caretaker who is capable of performing the consistent work of the good mirroring parent, now experienced as an object so intertwined in one's self as to be experienced as a *selfobject*, i.e., so close to one's self yet still an outside force under the self's control. Through many admiring-echoing-approving experiences, the self internalizes these ap-provals from the outside and begins to feel self-worth, self-value—the process of transmuting internalization. At the same time, in the ontogeny of the self another development takes place—the merger of the infant self with the parent who calms, soothes, and offers guidance and protection. This parent is experienced as a greater-than-life idealized figure (Kohut, 1977). Once internalized, this selfobject now takes its place in the infant's self as the self's experience of self-calming structure along with the other accre-tions from the internalization of the goals and values of one's idealized parents. The final form of the nuclear self is that of one pole, the pole of ambitions expressing through its talents and skills actions that, in fact, live up to the standards and values of one's poles of ideals. In self psychology terms, the self is pro-pelled by the tension arc that exists between one's pole of ideals and one's pole of ambitions (Kohut, 1977).

The model of the self is of service in establishing an empathic diagnosis. An empathic diagnosis must, to begin with, center on the particular self's capacity for adaptive action which reflects the integrity or deficiency in the self-pole of ambitions. Likewise, the diagnosis must uncover evidence for the functioning of the other pole of the self, the patient's ideals and standards for himself. Other self-functions that are crucial to assess include the self-observing function, the crucial capacity of the self to determine inner from outer experience which provides the basis for intro-spection and empathy for oneself. The self-observing function is necessary in the formation of a so-called therapeutic alliance be-tween patient and therapist.

The therapist must assess the overall posture of the self in a *developmental* continuum. To begin with, the therapist must de-termine whether the self is firm, cohesive, and, in the main, expe-riencing an overall sense of well-being. The cohesive self has ade-quate sources of self-worth and is capable of withstanding blows to its narcissistic endowment without decompensation (the expe-rience of disintegration anxiety and loss of integrity of the self that we call fragmentation). On the obverse side of the cohesion stands the immature, fixated self that is mirror-hungry or ideal-hungry. These immature selves seek out persons, or surrogates of persons such as drugs, to perform these archaic selfobject functions of reacting to them with total admiration or of exerting control or of being a source of calming. In contrast to the need of the cohesive self to be provided with warmth and admiration from a mature selfobject who temporarily offers invigoration to a flagging self, people with immature or deficient selves enter into relationships that hopefully will finally replenish their empty selves with the sustenance they missed, i.e., to actually give them archaic mir-roring which they hope to internalize so as to form the structures of self-value they are missing.

The result of the empathic diagnostic phase is to finally arrive at a profile of the scrutinized self. We wish to be able to conclude that the self we have observed is either a basically cohesive self, with self-observing functions intact, or a self that is deficient in one or many self functions, such as a mirror-hungry or ideal-hungry self, an overall enfeebled or empty self (devoid of self-worth). We have already noted that these enfeebled selves are ordinarily especially vulnerable to rebuff, rejections, or losses, to which they may respond with even more massive experiences of loss of esteem and decompensate into the panic reactions of fragmentation or the blind objectless rage that we call narcissistic rage. Especially important as a precipitant to the collapse of the enfeebled self is the breakup or rupture of an archaic self/selfobject bond, i.e., a relationship with a figure in one's environment who performs archaic mirroring functions or has become a target for idealization, akin to a relationship with an idealized selfobject from one's past. (The diagnosis arrived at in this phase of therapy is not a DSM-III diagnosis; it is a diagnosis of the functions or malfunctions of the self.)

THE THERAPEUTIC DIAGNOSIS

Directly after the work of the empathic diagnosis is completed, the therapist, on the basis of his findings, is able to establish goals for his therapy. The goals will then proceed from the empathically derived diagnoses of the shape of the self, and the integrity or deficiency of its functioning. These are the only considerations in arriving at a prescription for the necessary therapeutic intervention. Thus, for example, in a patient who is found to be experiencing symptoms of a pervasive lack of worth and is highly reactive to losses and rebuffs but who on the other hand is achieving well in his profession and has a capacity for self-observing, the recommended therapy would be psychoanalysis. The cure would consist of the attempt to form a curative transference relationship and hopefully end with a filled-out self that has overcome the deficiencies and rebuffs of the past.

In another instance in which the self of the patient reveals that there is now and has always been a deficiency in mirroring in the person's past, which has resulted in an acute or chronic experience of emptiness and loneliness and overall inadequacy in life, the prescription might be that of advising supportive therapy. This diagnosis is based on the findings that the observed self is in frank disequilibrium and requires immediate repair. The disequilibrium may take the form of a massive and prolonged loss of esteem, such as after a loss of a loved one. In other instances, the disequilibrium might take the form of a fragmentation or panic state, again requiring instant repair. If the patient's central lesion is the capacity to experience self-worth, the goals of the supportive therapy will be to develop a self/selfobject relationship in which the therapist's functions will center on *being* a mirroring selfobject, akin to the archaic selfobject of childhood. Similarly, in those instances of disequilibrium in which the self of the patient is in need of guidance, calming, and soothing, the therapist's functioning will be to form a self/selfobject bond in which he functions as a leader and calmer and offers himself as a noncritical target for idealization.

In those instances in which there does not exist a need for the curative action of a psychoanalysis or the patient's self is not capable of going through an analysis for a variety of reasons *but* the patient does have adequate self-observing capacities, this patient can be helped to form important insights into his fixations, the basis for understanding his experiences of the past in the present. This therapeutic approach, that of so-called psychoanalytic psychotherapy or sector psychotherapy, rests on the establishment of a basic self/selfobject transference, which, however, in distinction from the approach of psychoanalysis proper, does not become *the* object of the therapy. In sum to this point, a therapeutic diagnosis represents the therapist's summarization of the findings derived from his diagnostic sessions—the empathic diagnosis—now plugged into the appropriate psychotherapy.

Those patients whose empathic diagnosis reveals that their selves are now in disarray—i.e., they are in frank disequilibrium, either depressed or fragmented, and cannot now or perhaps in the future ally themselves with the therapist to understand their intrapsychic dilemma—should be advised to enter into supportive therapy. This approach, perhaps best referred to as sustaining therapy, has as its goals the restitution of self-equilibrium through the medium of a self/selfobject transference bond.

In other patients who present with a specific psychological problem and whose selves are not currently in disarray and have intact self-observing functions, the appropriate therapeutic diagnosis is to recommend psychoanalytic psychotherapy. The goals of this approach are to alleviate, through insight and the self-enhancing of a basic self/selfobject transference bond, a specific psychological symptom such as a work inhibition. In these patients, the therapist must determine, as previously noted, that their selves are intact, apart from the problem area for which they seek relief, and that, therefore, they do not require psychoanalysis. The therapist, with this diagnosis, predicts that after the symptoms are alleviated the patient will be in psychic equilibrium, albeit capable of further symptom-formation. The methods that are important in this approach are those of the establishment and maintenance of the self/selfobject transference with the utilization of interpretation aimed at giving the patient an insight into the underlying aspects of the symptom. In this therapeutic approach, the therapist and the patient join—in their therapeutic alliance—in countless investigations aimed at exposing the roots of the defined dilemma so as to ultimately ferret out the past in the present. As will be elaborated in the chapters on the process of insight psychotherapy, this therapeutic approach does *not* involve a focus on the exposition of the transference onto the therapist as its method of alleviation of distress.

Finally, the therapeutic diagnosis that recommends psychoanalysis is based on the empathic diagnosis of a self-distress or characterological distress in which the self is in a pervasive and repetitious state of distress which will *not* be alleviated by the relief of a selfobject bond alone or by solving through insight a current and specific psychological dilemma. To recommend psychoanalysis, the therapist must have gathered the data which demonstrate that the patient can ally himself with the therapist and can, without suffering unremitting fragmentation, undergo the experience of being on the couch in the so-called therapeutic regression of living through a transference neurosis.

The following vignettes of case histories represent instances of typical psychotherapeutic situations in which an empathic diagnosis of the state of the self is followed by a therapeutic diagnosis of the appropriate therapeutic modality for the patient.

Case 1

Mr. L. B., a 48-year-old lawyer, came to his initial session complaining of increasing disharmony in his marriage. His wife told him that he was emotionally distant from her, withdrawing into his interests in sports by watching television or by going to athletic events without her. Although he corroborated her version of their difficulties that he did indeed stay away from contact with her for long periods, he was markedly distressed over her threat that they should separate if he could not control his distance-making behavior. He immediately launched into a long list of complaints about his wife's intolerance of his relationship with his childhood caretakers and of the sports activities in which he engaged with his children and she did not participate. His next associations were to her tyrannizing of him through her depriving him of their children's contacts with him—"she's always pulling them away from me"—and her frequent criticism of him: "She really has a temper—can say anything—and she can get real upset but if I say anything it's terrible and she'll fight." After a long exposition of his wife's harassment of him and his impotent attempts at fending off her malevolence, he began to spontaneously associate to his childhood:

> My wife scares me—although I'd never tell her that—when she starts with this separation talk. You know, my mother died when I was born. Things were bad for me when I was a kid. My father didn't know what to do with me. Apparently I was in an orphanage for a while, then his sister who was already pretty old took care of me for the next several years. I don't remember her much. My mother's sister took me from

her when I was three; apparently I was being neglected. I *know* I'm sensitive over separations.

The therapist replied: "Well, you put it together very nicely. Your distress is becoming understandable. What is not easy to understand is what the withdrawal is all about. We have to understand what's making you seek distance from your wife." The patient responded:

Well, I see a lot of things that she doesn't see herself. I see her say things and do things that weave webs that she doesn't even know she's doing I don't think because she's really basically a good person. But for instance, with my family, there has been almost a 100% cutoff from my family because her family is so small that when anything comes up during the year, any holidays, it's always with her family, because if we don't go, there is nothing. At the same time, even though my family is a little bit larger, because it's not my *real* mother, it's my aunt who raised me . . . that she's just . . . it has . . . she has made me see very painfully that all she is is my aunt. She's not my mother. I don't give her Mothers' Day presents, I don't even give her birthday presents anymore. Everything for her kids—they were my cousins who I grew up with in the same house . . . when they don't invite us to something, she always points it out. She brings it out, and she makes my family into nothing. The other day, I just had a little bit of insight. I got to tell her that they may not be perfect, but that's the only one I got, and she's taking that away. She's cut that off. She's cut my family off, but I can't say she's done it, because she'll turn . . . and there'll be a tremendous, tremendous argument because she'll turn it around and say, "Well, you're just living in a dream world. It's not yours. They don't love you." My aunt took a lot of the crap with me, all my whole life, and she made some mistakes, you know. If she would have been a little nicer, maybe I wouldn't have had such a hard life. But she wasn't that bad. You know, she was who she was. She was a simple woman, and I really love her, but it's been cut off. I mean, I can't treat her like I want to treat her because she'll say, "What are you making a fool of yourself for? What are you putting yourself out for?" That's what she's going to say. I can't tell it to her. There'll be a tremendous argument.

In relation to his father, Mr. L. B. stated:

> My father, I haven't . . . I haven't seen in almost a year. My wife made me a big birthday party last June at Sox Park. They have a place behind the bleachers at Sox Park called the Patio, and it was a surprise party. She invited my father and his wife, and they wouldn't come. It was too hard to get there. Well, I figured that's the last time. He didn't show up to my graduation at high school. He didn't come to my first wedding, not to my birthday. That's it! I mean, how many times can you take crap? You know. So I just . . . the only time he used to call me was when he needed something anyhow, so the hell with that. Well, my aunt wasn't like that.

In the second and third interviews, Mr. L. B. continued to reveal in his behaviors and associations, not with awareness of their identification with the past, that his current interactions with his wife at times resembled his previous interactions with his aunt. In relation to his wife, he again emphasized that she complained of his ongoing need to divorce himself from her each night or, even after a social engagement, to closet himself in the den and immerse himself in an athletic program on television. In relating these vignettes, Mr. L. B. made it clear that there was a ritualistic aspect to his nocturnal behaviors. The interviewer responded by encouraging him to "put this behavior under the microscope and freely associate any thoughts or memories of a similar nature to this nocturnal behavior." His associations went as follows:

> Well, I did do something secret at night when I was a kid. I had a radio which I took to bed. I always had trouble going to sleep at night, I was a scared kid. I had to sleep on this

sleeping porch and it was lonely. Also, my real mother's picture was on the buffet table in the dining room, her eyes were always on me following me wherever I went. When I was four or five, I remember going to a funeral and seeing the body in the open casket. We went to visit the family afterwards. No one told me the dead lady had a twin so that when we got to this house and she greeted us, I was petrified. Well, my aunt, she was always mad at me for going to sleep with that radio which kept going all night. Once she woke me up and had me stand at attention until 2:00 A.M. I used to go to sleep with that little radio next to me all the time.

Apart from these distresses in his interactions with his spouse, the patient related that he had been quite successful in many areas of life—as an attorney, in his relations with friends, and in leadership activities in the community.

The empathic diagnosis. As noted, the empathic diagnosis represents a description of what is currently amiss in the self of the patient. As the therapist gathers the patient's interview behaviors and the patient's description of his self in reaction to various human and other encounters, he (the therapist) is led to a description of the operations of the self.

In the case of Mr. L. B. described above, the empathic diagnosis was as follows: Mr. L. B. had a self disorder which emerged most prominently in his encounters with his wife. In these encounters he would undergo a self-transformation in which she was experienced as an archaic selfobject, akin to his aunt-mother. Also in these encounters he would become a subservient youngster to his maternal selfobject. When these transformations were completed, Mr. L. B. was immersed in an archaic idealized selfobject transference in which he experienced ineptitude and loneliness. In his current transference to his wife as in the original self/selfobject relationship of his past, Mr. L. B. defended himself from the real and fantasied malevolence by stonewalling his environment and pursuing substitute activities for the human interactions that were painful. The empathic diagnosis, then, in this case needed to include the description of the self disorder being limited, for the most part, to the interaction with the patient's wife, in which the patient experienced what is best referred to as a defense transference: the patient was in an archaic self/selfobject transference bond in which the selfobject transference figure, the wife, was defended against by the patient who adopted those defenses which, in the past, had maintained his self in equilibrium.

Apart from the self-constraints experienced by Mr. L. B. with his spouse, his life was productive and he felt himself fulfilled. He was a partner in his law firm, his expertise being in real estate law. He had been an accomplished athlete in water sports in his youth and had continued his interests in these activities by coaching a YMCA team of youngsters interested in swimming.

The other aspects of the interview material that are essential to recognize are the data that reveal the patient's capacity and/or need to enter into an investigative (or alliance) dyad as contrasted to those patients who cannot enter into an alliance and require direction or help. Another necessary element to be evaluated in the interview data is the patient's capacity to self-observe—to stand apart from himself as it were and view the internal experiences of his self. These two capacities—the capacity to join with a therapist *and* the capacity to observe one's self—to view one's problems as intrapsychic and interpersonal are crucial in the therapeutic diagnosis, providing the basis for what is necessary and possible for psychic relief.

In the case of Mr. L. B., he demonstrated that he could enter into a study of his self with the therapist and that he had sufficient capacity for self-observation. The data for this emerged during several interactions in which he took a suggestion of the therapist and worked with it by bringing forth associations from his past. For example, in the first interview, the therapist suggested that from the data Mr. L. B. sounded frightened over leaving his practice over the weekend. He commented to the therapist:

> Yes, I have anxieties over separation, probably has to do with my mother dying before I was born. This weekend be-

fore I saw you, I suddenly felt panicked over not going to the office over the entire weekend. I hit myself in the head and I said, "You know, you damn fool, it will be there tomorrow." I get this buildup of tension inside me, unrelated to the real world.

However, Mr. L. B.'s description of the situation with his wife showed a marked absence of insight into his experience, so that his turmoil with her was understood as being related only to her *literal* power over him, not his *experience* of her.

The therapeutic diagnosis. The indications for a specific therapy come from the empathic diagnosis, which informs the therapist of the nature and extent of the self-disarray and the capacities or deficits of the self that will allow for a particular therapeutic modality. In the case of Mr. L. B. his self-difficulties were limited, in the main, to an inhibition of his self, which in itself reflected an instance of an archaic transference. In other areas of his life he had achieved well, so there was no evidence of a pervasive disturbance affecting all areas of his life. Further, there was no evidence of impending or frank disarray. Thus, the therapeutic diagnosis was to advise psychoanalytic psychotherapy, indicated by the absence of crisis or disarray—the usual indications for supportive psychotherapy—and the absence of pervasive difficulties in many areas of life especially human encounters—the usual indication for psychoanalysis. Moreover, the positive indications were quite clear in this case: a circumscribed area of self disorder without fragmentations in a person who had the capacity for self-observation and who could enter into an alliance to study his difficulties.

Case 2

Ms. C. M., a 41-year-old linotypist, was referred for relief of her depression, which developed after a mastectomy had been performed three-and-a-half months previously. Her initial comments were that she was now "a helpless person" and of very little use to anyone, especially her mother with whom she now lived. As she stated in her first interview:

It's ugly! And I'm ugly! Oh boy, I'm just so tired. This chemotherapy just knocks me out. I'm just not able to get off that couch for hours. When you add to that tiredness the awful, awful nausea, it's quite a party. I can't fight my feelings. I look in the mirror—to me I'm ugly. I can't fight it. (*cries*) When you have a breast missing, it's not pretty. And I'm so tired all the time. At first it didn't bother me.

My mother is a very demanding 80-year-old. The last three months have been different around the house. I'm used to doing everything around the house and I suppose my mother still thinks I'm as strong and as reliant as ever. Of course, half the time I'm on the couch. She'll never change. She doesn't believe in psychiatrists. (*chuckles*)

Cancer has been a killer in our family. The doctor said after surgery that it was in the lymph nodes and he said I have five to 10 years. I thought, it's all over now! I've had two deaths in the family recently. My mother had two knees replaced one year ago. She's OK now.

I'm afraid to go back to work [lithography]. I get exhausted after one hour. I am big-busted. Now I feel I should hide, now it's not there. Now I sit and sleep. (*cries*) I don't like that. (*cries*) I like to be doing things. Always to have people reminding me that I'm goofing up, that I shouldn't be laying around, that hurts. I'm used to helping.

We've had tragedies recently. My nephew got killed by a car as he was fixing a flat tire. My sister had a bilateral mastectomy three years ago. My brother died when I was 15. (*cries*) We were like twins. When he died, a part of me died. (*cries*) Will you look at me crying like this? My dad died two years after my brother of a heart attack. I'm acting like a crybaby. (*prolonged crying*)

In response to the interviewer's inquiries about her present situation, Ms. C. M. replied:

I live with my mother. She's the ruler of the roost, whatever mother says goes. She is a good woman whose expectations I cannot live up to. I very much want to leave but she is

80 years old. If anything happens, I would blame myself for the rest of my life.

In the second session she related:

> My mother's a demanding woman—everything to her standards and now! Can you imagine, she calls *me* lazy! I'm not up to heavy house cleaning. I can't leave her and justify it in my mind. She is hard to take. Everything has to be her way or else. She can't understand my wishes for my freedom. But I can't leave. If I left and something happened—if she broke a leg, got a heart attack, or whatever—I'd be struck with guilt for my life. I have to stay there. I'll have to wait for her to die before I can live.

In answer to the question about the beginnings of her attitudes towards responsibility, Ms. C. M. said:

> I was always a tomboy. I couldn't stand the little girl stuff, it made me feel hemmed in. My mother always wanted me to be the little girl but I couldn't stand it and I still can't. I can't stand these clothes, those frills, those manners. It's not that I don't like men, just that I don't feel the attraction to be with them physically. I respect 'em, I work with 'em. At home and at work I guess I always feel I *have* to be the responsible one.

The empathic diagnosis. Ms. C. M. was at this point immobilized. In retrospect, her oncologist and she could now see that her lassitude and diminished self-esteem had been growing since her mastectomy. Her capacity to feel comforted by her physicians, relatives, and friends was virtually nonexistent as she suffered all by herself. The empathic diagnosis was that of an enfeebled self which was suffering with the pain of the precipitous loss of self-worth. She related this loss of self-value to the loss of an important aspect of her attractiveness (the breast), as well as to the loss of status as the responsible caretaker of her mother and the family home (loss of strength).

In the background were several issues related to the fixation of her self. One major self issue was her experience of herself as permanently bound to her archaic selfobject mother whose sustenance was required for her survival. The patient expressed this bond in the converse: it was her *mother* who needed *her* for her survival. The other issue centered on her fear of becoming manifestly receptive to her mother or anyone; her self-capacity to unfold dependency strivings was limited to symbolic and displaced situations where *she* did the nurturing. Her own wishes for mirroring or calming–soothing responses were clearly unpalatable, ostensibly tied up with memories of frustration and pain associated with those childhood states of need for a mirroring selfobject or an idealized selfobject. However, these were background issues at this point since the foreground was a self-in-disequilibrium, a self in a painful state of an acute loss of self-value.

The therapeutic diagnosis. The therapeutic diagnosis was for supportive psychotherapy, i.e., that this self needed shoring up, needed an infusion of worth through the medium of an archaic selfobject bond in which the patient hopefully would experience herself again as being of value. The therapeutic value of supportive psychotherapy is that the self, once it has joined in an archaic self/selfobject bond, experiences the cohesive power of the selfobject's admiration or calming or togetherness and regains its intactness. In the case of Ms. C. M. once the patient's self had regained its equilibrium, there might be a need on her part to enter into a psychotherapeutic investigation of her chronic self-distresses in her relationship with her mother and in other areas of her life; but at this moment, the therapist and patient must concern themselves with the issue that was most compelling: a fragmenting self suffering with a precipitous loss of self-regard and in danger of even greater fragmentation and/or self-destructiveness.

Case 3

Ms. B. C. came for a consultation a few years after a previous analysis from which she had derived considerable benefit; she had married, had delivered two infants, and had acquired an attractive house which she had furnished well. In her first interview, however, she told of the inner experience which continued to distress her—the unremitting feeling of being unloved. As a result of these and other pervasive experiences all centering on inferiority, she found herself in each relationship and in each role she was in to be preoccupied with the possibility of an imminent outburst of criticism. These experiences, well known to her since childhood, were not alleviated during or after her previous analysis.

The patient's initial complaints were that she was experiencing a depression which had persisted for over six months. She was at that time in mourning for her father, dead for one year. She had given birth to her last child, her second, four months prior to the time she came for the consultation. At the time of her first interview, she was a slightly-built and fragile-appearing 32-year-old woman. She related that she had been in both analysis and psychotherapy since she was 20. Her mother, who died of breast cancer when she was a senior in college and who, since her high-school days, had been ill with a depression, had become more depressed since Ms. B. C. entered college. The patient, reacting to her mother's distress, could not study as she had herself become depressed and agitated, and so she arranged for psychotherapy. Directly after her mother's death, Ms. B. C. went into analysis, which lasted until her marriage when she was 25 and was terminated with "good results." One of the good results was that she was able to socialize more easily and overcome her fear of an intimate relationship with a man. The analysis, as she said, was "all about my oedipus complex, my wish to dethrone my mother."

The major data of her background that she came to reveal were that she had had a life of tragedy from her earliest memories—a life without the uplifting of an adequate mirroring presence through all of her development. Her mother, she recalled, was unable to calm her at any time. She became, in fact, so distressed over her mother's ministrations that she cried and became agitated when her mother did attempt to hold her. The patient was told innumerable times that her first years were marked by being a colicky infant and that she had been considered a candidate for surgery for this condition in her first year of life (probably due to a pyloric stenosis). Ms. B. C. never experienced her mother as a source of warmth or of nurturance; she would always be vigilant and fearful around her mother lest her mother find something amiss in her behavior and become critical.

Thus, the major instigator of Ms. B. C.'s lifelong psychic distress was revealed to be her experience of her mother as an imprisoner. Although she could and did clamor, seemingly for attention, throughout her life and in her analysis, the capacity to receive and, therefore, ultimately accrete a self-structure of self-calming and self-soothing was always interfered with by the prospect of the fearful dismissal. She was restricted, therefore, to empty complaining—complaining without the appropriate action of obtaining relief—that she was not being given the proper attention; but actually, she restricted herself to being on the outside in all her relationships, a victim of the unconscious equation of closeness being equal to imprisonment.

It is, of course, no surprise that she never came to her mother for aid, fearing either coldness or criticism, and so she became an isolate in her own home, always lonely, always feeling cold. She was also agitated in school and in most interpersonal encounters, could not sit for any length of time, and, therefore, could not comfortably sink into books, movies, or conversations. On the other hand, she was not totally without stimulation; it was just that there was limited capacity on her part to unfold herself and be adequately lifted up—physically or emotionally. The stimulation she did get was from her mother, a former piano teacher, who ran the house like a military installation with rules and fines until she became ill, when the patient was 12. Her other sibs, Ms. B. C. reported, were somewhat less awed or frightened by her mother, were less nervous than she; but the atmosphere in the house was cold for all. No one touched or hugged or kissed or, even more significantly, smiled at one another when mother was around.

Her father, towards whom Ms. B. C. felt more positively, was a warm person; he did show humor and he did try to engage her in her early teens in his sports—fishing and boating—to which she responded. However, in the first several years of her life, he was not home a great deal; he was away on business, coming home mainly on weekends. In later years, he took the entire family on fishing, boating, and hiking trips, in which she participated with pleasure, but always as one of the family; she did not have an exclusive relationship with her father. Stated more simply and more to the point, her father did not function as a major selfobject presence. He remained in her self-experience as an idealized persona from afar who did not utilize his powers to teach, guide, or even influence her destinies in all of her activities from early learning experiences to choice of friends or college or marriage, and so forth. We are, of course, reporting on what the father was for this patient; that he might have been more of a leader or calmer in the family we can only surmise, since with him, as with her mother, Ms. B. C. was vigilant and, therefore, not able to engage in a relationship.

Ms. B. C.'s experiences in secondary school paralleled those at home; she became superficially attached to a group of young women and practiced what she had perfected at home—to be the accommodating friend and never to display self-needs. Unfortunately for her learning, her capacity to "take in" from her instructors and books was interrupted (and this continued until her analysis); she did not enter into a dialogue with teachers or authors. In high school, she neither dated nor engaged in any social activities. One reason was that since early high school days, her mother became more and more isolated and was diagnosed as suffering with a depression. The patient and her siblings were subject for several years to minimal supervision since the mother was chronically depressed and received regular psychotherapy from the time the patient was 15. Ms. B. C.'s home situation was so depressing that neither she nor her siblings ever brought friends into her house. When she was 18 and started college in her hometown, her mother's condition worsened, necessitating hospitalization. It was at this time that Ms. B. C. first started psychotherapy. In her senior year at college, it was discovered that her mother had cancer of the breast which had already widely metastasized. Her death, only one year after the discovery of cancer, was reacted to by the patient with a mixture of sadness and relief that the suffering was at an end. Her mother had not been able to receive any relief from her psychic and physical distresses for many years.

The patient's first analysis was, as has been previously noted, helpful to her in many ways. She became able to relate to men at her work. She had become an elementary school teacher—albeit with anxiety—and began going to group parties and dances. Her analyst, Ms. B. C. informed the therapist, had concentrated on her special feeling of competitiveness with her mother for her father's interest and had not focused on her childhood of isolation.

Ms. B. C. met her first beau at a dance and one month afterwards they married. She had great respect for his serious approach to life and devotion to ideals in his work and family ties. Her relationship to him had been, until her analysis, marred by her lifelong difficulty in receptivity. Although her husband had been somewhat reserved in his manner, the patient's barriers to being cherished were the major obstacle to their romantic involvement. In relating to her children, there had been a similar pattern of transference interference so that the patient could not experience the mergers of the parent-child bond and could only perform in a dutiful manner as wife and mother. Her equilibrium was disrupted after her first analysis when her father suddenly died of a cerebrovascular accident. She experienced this event as a catastrophe of aloneness, although she had seen him infrequently over the years since her mother's death. As she later came to understand, this event symbolized the end of any aspirations to achieve recognition of her archaic needs for merging; her father's death signified the end to any promise of a self/selfobject life with him or anyone else.

The empathic diagnosis. This patient revealed that she had been experiencing self-deficits throughout her life. Indeed, her previous analysis could not alter her self-state. Further, she revealed a capacity to form an alliance of goals, was able to articulate her experiences, and did not have an untoward reaction to the therapist's investigative comments.

The therapeutic diagnosis. The patient had a pervasive self-disorder requiring a self-transformation. The therapeutic diagnosis was that Ms. B. C. should have a psychoanalysis.

We will now proceed to the chapters on the work of psychotherapy. The first of these chapters will present the approaches in the
work of supportive psychotherapy for those patients whose specific empathic diagnoses of disequilibrium make it clear that this
modality is required.

4

The Supportive Psychotherapies

Supportive psychotherapy has as its goal the restoration of psychic equilibrium in those patients who are experiencing psychic disarray. Among this broad group of patients are those in the throes of an immobilizing depression, as well as those who are experiencing massive anxiety with fragmentation of the self. The essential psychological malfunction in these reactions of disequilibrium from whatever source is the loss or diminished functioning of the self-mechanisms that maintain the cohesion of the self. Among these vital self-functions are: the repression barrier against emergence of disruptive archaic affects and drives; the capacity to perceive and test reality; the capacity to synthesize thoughts and feelings without derailing; and the self-capacity to maintain experiences of worth in the face of repudiations and/or separations.

The central ingredient in supportive psychotherapy is the development of the self/selfobject tie or transference between patient and therapist. The self/selfobject bond will of course reflect the self-needs of the individual patient in harmony with the empathic therapist so that the unit in one instance will unfold as a mirroring bond, while in other instances the self/selfobject dyad will be based on an idealized parent model. Whatever the differences in the self/selfobject unit, the symptoms of psychic disequilibrium are relieved when the patient's self becomes bonded with the therapist-as-selfobject.

In order for the patient requiring supportive psychotherapy to enter into a therapeutic bond, there must be sufficient trust in human encounters, the capacity to feel safe in unfolding to another the dilemmas and distresses that have evoked the psychic disarray. The next requirement for the patient in supportive therapy is his ability to transfer onto the therapist selfobject features derived from his selfobject background that are vitally needed to restore the patient's malfunctioning self.

In those patients who are unable to form the requisite self/selfobject bond, the difficulty at times lies in a "defense against the transference." This resistance reflects the association in the patient's self between human contact and the danger of rejection. The rejection may be in the form of a feared rebuff or it may take the form of fantasied abandonment at the hands of a significant human object or selfobject. Another resistance to the formation of the therapeutic bond lies in the emergence in the patient of a *"defense transference"* which interferes with the required selfobject transference needed for relief of the psychological distress. Defense transference refers to the process in which the patient unconsciously transfers onto the therapist the salient features of the disappointing and/or malevolent parent(s) and the simultaneous revival of experiences and behaviors of the archaic defenses in the patient's self *against* this parental malevolence. The patient in a defense transference reenacts the past, holding back or fighting against his or her revived involvement with the therapist-as-parent (Daniels, 1976; Gitelson, 1952, 1962; Schlessinger & Robbins, 1983). The patient in a "defense-against-the-transference" will have difficulty in engaging the therapist in *any* manner; interaction with and trust of humans are at a minimum.

From the point of view of the therapist performing supportive therapy, there are a variety of tasks to be accomplished. The initial task is to empathically diagnose the state of the uncohesive self requiring supportive measures. Following the initial therapeutic diagnosis, the therapist uncovers which therapeutic posture is required for *this* patient, i.e., which selfobject functions it is necessary to restore in the self-under-observation to establish equilibrium. In a nutshell, the therapist is to be a selfobject-in-function to his patient's self; this is the central feature of any supportive psychotherapy. It also is a source of resistance in some therapists at some times since it requires action and other activities that are difficult to perform or are unacceptable behaviors to these psychotherapists. (The resistances and stresses of the therapist will be addressed a little further on in this chapter.) The selfobject function of mirroring, for example—the quintessential activity in supportive therapy—requires that the therapist function as an empathic authority figure who serves covertly and *overtly* as an endorser of the patient's self and thereby elevates the patient's esteem once the patient invests the therapist with parental-like status (transference).

The activities of the therapist when he becomes an idealized parent selfobject are those of the leader who at times calms and soothes, while at other times he directs and advises and restrains to institute or maintain self-cohesion. And when the therapist functions as a selfobject with twinshiplike qualities, he attempts to infuse into the contact with the patient those special features of *essential sameness* which are the essence of the twinship bond.

In each instance of supportive psychotherapy, the empathic diagnosis of the self and its needs for cohesion will determine the necessary selfobject posture. The selfobject requirements will change, at times even within the space of a therapy session, so that the therapist must be alert through his empathic assessment in the therapy to the fluctuating selfobject needs of his patient (although a dominant profile of the self/selfobject unit is usual throughout the therapy). These latter considerations of the uniqueness of the supportive measures that need to be employed eliminate the notion of supportive therapy as a monolithic psychotherapeutic approach that emphasizes "managing" each patient's life or aims, without the data of the self-needs, which are required so as to determine the specific selfobject functions necessary in each case.

To return to the stresses and resistances of the therapist, it is important to emphasize at the outset that being a supportive psychotherapist is indeed difficult work. It requires of the therapist activities often unfamiliar to a therapist. To begin with, the supportive therapist not only has to *adopt* a particular posture (to be the mirror, idealized parent, etc.), but he then also has to *exhibit* the required and specific selfobject functions. Each session and each interaction require that the therapist not only "see" but also "be" a selfobject in some particular manner who performs a relevant selfobject function. The supportive therapist is therefore on call in each session and has to perform, in contrast to the therapist in other therapies whose task is to follow the material and study with the patient different aspects of the psyche in an attempt to gain insight into the patient's nuclear conflicts.

Therapists differ widely in their self-makeup and thus in their capacities to "be" one or other of the model selfobject constellations. Further, therapists differ within themselves at *different times* in their capacities to perform these vitally needed selfobject functions. Also, therapists vary in their abilities to perform different selfobject functions due to the intrusion of their own transferences onto their patients. Finally, therapists exhibit differences in their capacities to perform in selfobject functions as a result of current stresses in their own lives. The psychotherapist who is in the midst of major stresses, enervated from overwork, or in the midst of a mourning state has great difficulty in functioning as a supportive figure who, regardless of his self-state, has to *be* a selfobject and turn away from his enervation of mourning to center on his patient's self. In these instances of the therapist harboring his own self-needs or struggling with an enfeebled self, the capacity for empathy is limited, as is the capacity to be the target of a transference and have to respond to the patient's self-needs which may be less (at least as experienced by the therapist) than the therapist's difficulties.

The interferences with the therapist's selfobject functioning as a selfobject that come from his self-development consist of those self-fixations which would make it difficult for the therapist to "be" one or another of the selfobject models. Being able to "be" a mirroring figure requires the capacity to experience the patient's nurturing needs without discomfort, which itself is a reflection of a background in which mirroring needs were responded to empathically and with compassion. Another necessary element in the self of the mirroring therapist to permit him to function as a selfobject is that he have a minimum of his own selfobject needs. The therapist who is himself—currently (temporary) or chronically—in need of nurturance cannot *easily* empathize with the self of a patient caught up with mirroring needs. The therapist who is caught up with his own needs may, of course, also turn to the *patient* for those mirroring needs in addition to being unable to recognize the patient's self-state of need. A final element that is an impediment to the therapist's functioning as a selfobject is the conflict in *values* that appears in some therapists over the task of being a selfobject in supportive therapy. Functioning as a selfobject is experienced by some therapists as deviating from the generally accepted model of the therapist in the psychoanalytic and psychotherapeutic arenas as a blank screen onto which the patient projects his or her unconscious complex. It seems to us that the important maxim here lies in the understanding that the supportive psychotherapist proceeds with the work of restoring the self of his patient in the most efficacious manner. At times this amounts to performing selfobject functions for a self that, while it is dismantled, is paralyzed. With the aid of the human encounter of the therapist-as-selfobject, this self *can* be restored to equilibrium, a worthwhile mission. In other forms of psychotherapy, the therapist does not ordinarily adopt a particular selfobject posture since the goal of restoring a self-in-disarray is not involved. However, in all instances of psychotherapy of any kind, the patient who experiences disequilibrium from any avenue may require the therapist to perform, even temporarily, selfobject functions to restore psychic equilibrium. Thus, in the midst of a psychoanalysis, the analyst is called on to "be" a selfobject if his patient requires support during an episode of disequilibrium, such as a death in the family.

THE COURSE OF SUPPORTIVE PSYCHOTHERAPY

There is a modal course in many cases of supportive psychotherapy. The course may be divided into four phases: 1) The establishment of rapport; 2) the defense transference, when present; 3) the formation of the self/selfobject bond and the activities of the therapist; 4) the termination.

1. The Establishment of Rapport

In all cases of psychotherapy, the therapist's first obligation to his patient is to establish a climate of safety, a haven where the patient may unfold his troubles. The therapist does this by his own equanimity, which will convey the message that the milieu of therapy offers repose to the troubled self of the patient. The therapist conveys this message further by his initial posture of concentration on the patient and his woes. From the beginning to the end of therapy, the interaction is always a monologue, never a dialogue. The rapport is aided further by the therapist's manner during the initial data gathering and throughout the therapy: he is not intrusive; he is unruffled; his manner is neutral but pleasant.

2. The Defense Transference

The defense transference as previously described becomes manifest in the beginning of any form of psychotherapy. It represents the patient's investment in the therapist of the important qualities of significant and disappointing or feared parental selfobjects to which the patient will respond by adopting a posture of defense against the power or malevolence of these selfobjects. For the patient to form a therapeutic bond requires that the defense transference be diminished sufficiently for the patient to develop a therapeutic mirroring or idealized or twinship bond. At times this defense transference will require interpretations to decrease its hold on the patient. At other times the patient's posture of the defense part of the defense transference is minimal and the defense transference becomes reduced through the repeated demonstrations of safety in the psychotherapy.

3. The Formation of the Self/Selfobject Bond

As the defense transference weakens or in those instances where the defense transference is minimal, the patient in disarray reveals his or her selfobject needs to the therapist. At times the communication is through behaviors, inside and outside the office, showing the need for soothing through manifest agitation or through episodes of mini-fragmentation. As the therapy continues and the patient enters into the specific selfobject transference, the work of selfobject bonding begins in earnest. Once into the functioning of the selfobject entity, the therapist expresses the supportive messages through words and gestures of the mirroring selfobject or the idealized parent selfobject or the message of the twinship selfobject.

4. The Termination

The work of supportive therapy ordinarily is terminated when the symptoms of psychic disequilibrium have been replaced by psychic peace in both the external behaviors and the inner experience (self-structure) of calm. There are, however, patients who cannot internalize the selfobject experiences they have received sufficiently for these to become self-structure. In these patients, the therapeutic self/selfobject bond must be maintained indefinitely in weekly, monthly, or p.r.n. contacts. With such patients, the therapist counts it as success that they have achieved a self/selfobject bond in which they experience equilibrium and therefore can function in their various activities and roles. In these situations of so-called interminability, the therapist's diagnosis of the required lifelong support is made after attempts to terminate have failed and it is clear that the patient's capacity for internalization is not sufficient for separation from psychotherapy. One other aspect of supportive therapy comes about when it is clear that the patient who is no longer in frank disequilibrium continues to have symptoms of a malfunctioning psyche and is still unable to enter into a variety of activities without circumscribed anxiety or shame. At this juncture, the therapist is now able to direct the patient into intensive psychotherapy of either the sector approach of insight psychotherapy or the broader goals of psychoanalysis (see Chapter 3).

CASE 1

A 41-year-old woman, Ms. C. M.,* sought relief for a depression which enveloped her self shortly after a mastectomy for breast cancer. She related the depression to the change in her appearance and also the change in her ability to work without excessive fatigue. In the initial interview she appeared immersed in grief but was able to describe the changes in herself and in her environment which, in her view, had dramatically altered her world. As she entered the room, she walked slowly and with embarrassment to the assigned chair; she had a dazed look on her face. She was wearing jeans and a polo shirt. Although everything about her person was neat, there was no attempt in her grooming to be decorative; for example, her hair was cut short and severe about her rotund face and she wore no makeup. Her entire body was slumped over as she sat; her face was downcast and her eyes did not meet those of the therapist for many minutes in the first interview.

Ms. C. M.'s initial comments were that she had experienced a profound twofold change in her self-view after her breast surgery. She was not prepared for the alteration in her self-appreciation and she was not prepared for the massive fatigue which she began to experience. As she related these changes, she cried and told of her inability to keep her thoughts together over the three months since her mastectomy. She said that she was so caught up with grief that she could not stop crying nor could she overcome her fatigue and get off the couch where she hibernated for hours.

In her first interviews Ms. C. M. described her experience of "ugliness" after the mastectomy. She stated that her recuperation was prolonged and filled with sadness and psychomotor retardation, which were so uncharacteristic of her. She then associated to

---

*See Chapter 3, pp. 52–55 for initial data gathering.

her 80-year-old mother and the difficulty her mother had in accepting her daughter's infirmity.

Mrs. C. M.'s next associations were to her lifelong history of being the "masculine" caretaker of her mother since her early adolescence when her father, a middle-aged trolley car conductor, suddenly died at work from a heart attack. However, long before that time she had established a self-pattern of being the "tough kid" with her family and friends. At this point in the history and in the interaction in the interview, there was no information about the mother's selfobject functioning. Did the mother perform easily and consistently as a mirroring selfobject in her responses to the developing youngster? Did she calm and soothe through bodily contact and how frequently? Or, as the data might imply, did she turn away from these selfobject nurturant functions so that her child equated early in life receptiveness and decorativeness with activities and self-states to be shunned? Since her early days Ms. C. M. felt uneasy with feminine clothing and any emphasis on being passively decorative. Instead, she was always given to activity; the rowdier, the better. She always played with boys and always played the sports that were ordinarily reserved for boys and men.

Her social life became confined, as the years went on, to being her mother's chauffeur and companion, especially since her father passed away. She described herself as a "loner" but she had always had extensive interactions with her sister (eight years her senior) and her sister's children as well as her mother. Her father was a man she knew very little. He had come from a northern European country early in his life and had always felt distant from the family and from his environment, staying away from most people. Ms. C. M. recalled pleasant experiences with him when they did household chores such as installing storm windows or chopping up the firewood.

The empathic diagnosis focused on Ms. C. M.'s self in disequilibrium, reacting to the surgery and the enforced passivity as an injury to her self-worth, thus ushering in a pervasive and prolonged loss of self-esteem, a depression. It should be pointed out that the patient experienced the self-state associated with the diagnosis of a major depression rather than the depressiveness of a narcissistic personality disorder (Val, Flaherty, & Gaviria, 1982; Val, Gaviria, & Flaherty, 1982). In a depression, the total self is enveloped in the pathognomonic trio of mental phenomena of loss of self-worth, grief, and psychomotor retardation. Also associated with a depression are the vegetative phenomena of anorexia, malaise, hypochondriasis, sleep disturbances, and gastrointestinal disturbances (e.g., constipation). The therapeutic diagnosis, the therapeutic prescription to alleviate this profound loss of self-value, was that Ms. C. M. required supportive psychotherapy. Of interest is that while she was taking the chemotherapy, she did, like all patients on chemotherapy, experience an enervation. However, this enervation has effects on patients that are quite idiosyncratic. To some it evokes a not-unpleasant lethargy, to others a distinctly unpleasant withdrawal.

The Course of the Psychotherapy

The patient's suffering centered on her experience of unattractiveness—she had become "ugly" and not simply due to a scar on her chest where once had been an attractive part of her body. As she related it, her lifelong involvement with her mother was contingent upon her performing as the caretaker and jack-of-all-trades. Her modal reaction to the anticarcinogen compounds of enervation in concert with the psychomotor retardation of her self-deflation combined to form an intense dysphoria when she came for therapy.

Phase 1: The Formation of Rapport

The therapeutic goal for Ms. C. M. was clear: to relieve the self-state of the massive experience of the loss of worth; or, to put it more operationally from the supportive psychotherapy point of view, to infuse the self with the selfobject charge of mirroring or calming necessary to reestablish self-worth and therefore self-cohesion. In supportive psychotherapy, as well as in psychoanalysis, there is at times a spontaneous unfolding of the therapeutic selfobject transference. In this case, Ms. C. M. stated her selfobject needs in the first session: her self was depleted of the essential experience of value. She required the infusion of worth from a selfobject who would offer this nurturance through the selfobject functions of mirroring and of becoming an idealizable target with whom she could merge, albeit temporarily, and accrue needed self-strength, and so the therapy began in the very first session.

In reacting to her first communication that she was "ugly" and experienced immobilizing lethargy, the therapist's responses as always were determined by the empathic observation of her painful inferiority. These comments and the subsequent association to the ungiving mother with whom she lived made it clear that the therapist's selfobject functioning had to be in the direction of a mirroring presence expressed in the therapist's listening and attending posture in order to diminish the painful self-state of ineptitude. The therapist demonstrated in his attentiveness and his verbal comments that he recognized and valued the experiences of the patient. In the first segment of the interview, these were the data:

Ms. C. M.: I can't fight it. I change my dressing in the morning and I have to look at it, I'm ugly. I say, What happened? Why am I so tired? Sure I'm *ugly* but what does that have to do with being tired all the time.

Therapist: What do you mean, sure you're ugly.

Ms. C. M.: I am, I think of what I lost. It's not pretty and what's the opposite of pretty. The only pretty thing I think is I'm alive and I have no cancer.

Therapist: The experience you had was that of the sudden painful feeling of losing your attractiveness.

In this sample, the therapist attempted to demonstrate his empathic recognition of the patient's self-state so that she feels someone understands her painful self-state and appreciates it.

Later the patient commented:

Ms. C. M.: My mother's a very demanding woman. She's 80 years old. It's hard for her to accept the fact that I'm sick. I've always been a hard-working person and since I've been living at home all my life I've been the man of the house doing all the work of keeping the place up. She can't accept it that I'm on the couch all the time, especially during the weeks I'm on chemotherapy. She wants me to run and jump and won't accept me the way I am now.

Therapist: That hurts your feelings I'm sure.

Even later she stated:

Ms. C. M.: I'm afraid to go back to work. I work as a linotype operator, I'm the only woman. I've seen all the men I usually work with in the hospital. I don't know why I don't want to face them. I suppose it's because I'm weak. I work around the house one hour, then I have to rest four hours. I can't stand it! (*cries*)

Therapist: You really feel quite different since the surgery. It takes time to get used to the changes and to recoup your strength.

In these early segments the therapist is attempting to show the patient his recognition of the unique experience she has had, suddenly feeling powerless and devalued. The hope at first is to establish an ambience of trust and appreciation so that she can unfold herself with safety. In this manner her experience of diminished value will be combatted by the therapist's communications of her value. In this interview she did respond to the mirroring by associating her disease with the loss of her brother and father:

Ms. C. M.: I don't like to be tired and bedridden and always be reminded by her [mother] that I should get moving and help her.

After this she cried and said: "How do you get me to cry so easily in here?"

Phase 2: The Establishment of the Self/Selfobject Bond

Already in the second session, the patient reported she felt "looser and less ugly." The therapist had made it clear in the first two sessions through his comments and his expressed interest that 1) the patient was not ugly and 2) she needed time to rest from the illness, the surgery, and the chemotherapy. In these initial sessions, Ms. C. M. expressed a great deal of sadness and cried deeply as she related her reactions to her malaise after the surgery and with the chemotherapy. A sample of these data is as follows:

Therapist: This is, of course, maybe the first time in your life you've had this special feeling by yourself—special feeling that you're not yourself—some loss of your normal esteem for yourself—your normal confidence. Is that true? Is this the first time?

Ms. C. M.: It's true—I haven't felt very confident or raring to go, getting everything done. Now I don't have any get-up and go. All I want to do is sit and sleep. Of course, when I do get interested in something . . . like I get interested in my roses, working in the yard, then the day goes by without any problem. Once I'm interested in something, fine, but until I get interested in something I think only a time bomb can get me motivated.

Therapist: So I think your mind is giving you a message that needs to be listened to—that you really do need time—to feel repaired. It's clear that this is a vital time for you, to allow yourself to hang back until you do feel more robust. But it's not easy for you. . . . That makes you feel sad right away, the whole idea that you need to withdraw for a while.

Ms. C. M.: (*nods*) I don't like that. I like being out doing things. And to be always tired, and always having people remind me, "Oh, my God, can't you move, are you always tired?" I think that, in itself. . . .

Therapist: Hurts your feelings, doesn't it? (*she nods*)

Ms. C. M.: I'm used to being needed and ready and able to do everything, and now I can't do it.

Therapist: You're not used to yourself being needy.

Ms. C. M.: No, no, I'm not. I'm used to being very independent . . . and still the tears. . . . What makes me cry?

Therapist: It's important to be in a place where you can feel safe to express yourself.

Ms. C. M.: My sister told me I should take notes. (*laughs*) She said she might need some help, too, after the loss of her son—her youngest son.

The therapist in this interaction is already functioning as a mixed selfobject who gives approval to the patient's outpouring of emotions as well as attempts to calm her through declaring to her that she is a valued person and that she needs to retire from activity until she feels safe to return to an active life.

As mentioned several times in previous sections, the therapist's selfobject functioning is the cornerstone of supportive therapy. Another cardinal precept of supportive therapy is the bond between the patient's self and the therapist as selfobject. The evidence for this merger is contained in the emergence of the state of equilibrium manifested by the diminution of the patient's symptoms of disequilibrium—those symptoms of anxiety or loss of worth that urged the patient to seek help.

The patient revealed a minor instance of a reequilibration of her self in the beginning of the second session:

Ms. C. M.: I've got more people telling me that I should solve my own problems.
Therapist: (*pause*) As we heard last session, for you to slow down and let someone listen to you is not easy.
Ms. C. M.: That's for sure. I've always been either a loner or plugging up a dike somewhere. I've been able to look at myself in the mirror this week. I don't feel so ugly. It helps to be here. I feel looser.

Her next association in this session was to talk of being tired at home and being tense.

Ms. C. M.: It's rough being at home, rough, rough. My mother is so demanding, she always wants her way. What she wants she wants *now*! She calls me lazy! It's only been three months since my surgery and she calls me lazy! About this house cleaning, she's been bugging me for weeks to start this house

cleaning and I can't do it. I spend an hour working and then I'll be four hours on the couch. (*cries*)
Therapist: You are tired, you are sad, and you need to stay away from hard work until you feel more robust.

In this manner she made it clear that the major loss of esteem was due to her loss of the support from the transformation of the particular self/selfobject dyad between her previous self of vigor and her selfobject mother's mirroring of this aspect of her self to the self in which she now found herself—an enfeebled shadow of her former robust self. The repair mission was now clear: the therapist must mirror her self of weakness lest she become more and more immobilized; hopefully, with this mirroring she will regain her vigor and proceed to resume her robust life.

And so she went on to tell of the injustices she suffered from her mother. The therapist's function as the mirroring selfobject was to agree with her experience of injustice and thus *validate* her experience of being abused. This validation in tandem with the continuing valuing of her need to hibernate would enhance her self-worth.

Now in the second session, the patient started to relate that she had been in two minds about continuing to stay with her mother. She would have liked to leave but her mother, now 80 years old, might have become ill or have had a traumatic fall which would have made her feel that she had been a bad daughter.

All of her wishes to maintain these ties with her mother were ascribed to guilt and the family's wishes for her to continue to live with her mother and keep her mother intact. The patient, on the other hand, was only conscious that she wished to leave but was hemmed in by responsibility and guilt:

Ms. C. M.: I can't leave her. She's 80. She might fall and then what? How much longer will it be before I get my freedom?
Therapist: You've been very special to her all these years, keeping her alive and well.
Ms. C. M.: What do I get out of it? Camaraderie and imprisonment. And it's always been that way. When I was 17, my dad

died. I had to step in and take over. My throat's so dry. Oh doctor, my goodness . . . a doctor getting me a glass of water. (*pause*) Yeah, well they all expect me to live with her. Why can't I have my own life? My mother pushed me into responsibility for the house, even before my father died. My mother's always pushing me. (*chuckles*) I used to always be a tomboy. She wanted me in dresses and skirts. I remember wearing a cowboy hat all my life as a kid.

Now, in the next session, she told of having an excellent week as far as her mood and self-cohesion were concerned, but then immediately associated to the tension in her home with her mother and her apparently newly found sensitivity (new as far as quantitative factors) to her mother's criticisms or lack of recognition:

Ms. C. M.: Being at home is turning into one big fight. My ma told me to take all my winter coats and bring them downstairs and then take her coats and put them into the back closet. I told her, "Goddamit, I live here too." She said, "What *do* you mean?" You see in her mind I'm just help. Then I start thinking about leaving. Then I start thinking of her age; what if she were alone and fell down? Oh, nuts! Does everyone think like this when they leave home?

Therapist: You've been responsible for her since you were a youngster.

Ms. C. M.: Yeah, but maybe I'm scared to be on my own. Maybe this stuff going on now is just obstruction I always get into. Now it's the cancer and the chemotherapy. When I tried to leave before, something always comes up. My ma says I'm too dependent on her. I don't know, I couldn't live if I knew she was sick by herself. Goddamit, she is a pistol. My ma is unhappy unless I'm working. But I just can't be the horse anymore. I need couch time each time I start to work. It's like I'm in the service. Orders, jump! It's caught up to me. My girlfriend says it's my decision to make. Either it's her [girlfriend] or it's my ma.

Therapist: Right now, it's important that no changes take place.

You're still convalescing and you need to stay in peace without making any changes.

Ms. C. M.: Everything revolves around my ma. I don't pass a day without thinking about her. My girlfriend wants me to leave. Should I leave?

Therapist: Everything must stay in place now.

Ms. C. M.: Everything is better but then my ma starts with her orders and commands and wham-bang! I'm in the war again! She's got to leave me up.

The patient, in increasingly better equilibrium, continued to focus on the central issue in her life: her fear of the possible rupture of her selfobject bond with her mother. The bond was being threatened at this time by her girlfriend and her own wishes to achieve some measure of autonomy. These wishes, one side of the conflict, were in balance with the other wishes to maintain permanent ties with the idealized selfobject mother. Thus the patient said, in the spirit of the youngster protesting the selfobject's tyranny *but* admitting that the selfobject has power:

> . . . my ma starts her orders and commands and wham-bang! I'm in the war again! She's got to leave me up.

In the same self-posture, Ms. C. M. stated that she never passed a day without thinking of her "ma."

The therapist's activity and position in maintaining equilibrium were determined by the need to keep the patient's self/selfobject ties intact at this time. The patient's fears of self-dissolution associated with the self/selfobject rupture of her bond with her mother were a potent source of fragmentation and needed to be appreciated. She revealed the depth of her ties clearly in this session, as well as the current threat to these ties. Further, she stated in another portion of this session that approximately one year prior to the discovery of her cancer and her breast surgery her girlfriend began "putting the screws on her" to force her to leave her mother. This psychic imbalance might have contributed either to the development of her breast tumor or to the growth of a previously existing breast mass. The therapist was called on to keep the peace, to maintain equilibrium by promoting the status quo. The actual therapeutic activity in this session was that of mirroring her achievements as a caretaker to her mother and being the idealized parent by exhibiting those functions of laying down a course of action: don't upset the apple-cart, stay in place for now.

In the following session, the patient announced that she was feeling more robust (the oncologist confirmed that her reports of malaise had diminished and she appeared more vigorous to herself and the oncology treating team) and that she needed little time on the couch in the two-week interval. She announced that she was, of course, still in combat with her mother but she was taking her mother with a "grain of salt. . . . I even told her to shut up when she started ordering me around this week."

At the end of this session, the patient, with much more vigor than she had previously shown, talked of having her own mobile home sometime in the future and said no one would be able to dissuade her.

It seemed clear that she had regained a self of vigor with the support of the psychotherapy, acknowledging that she needed rest, that she needed to stay in place with her mother, and above all that her wounded body self had value. Even though she could not perform at work and at home as she had previously, *she* was of worth. This correction in her self-balance helped her to regain equilibrium and secondarily allowed her to regain her position with her mother which was based on her being robust and in charge of the household. Being "on the couch" had threatened her valued position as her mother's valued hired hand and led to her fear of the self/selfobject bond rupture, which in turn led to her fear of abandonment.

Phase 3: Termination

In the final two visits, the patient related that she had come into better equilibrium and was going to return to work after a vacation in the south; her chemotherapy was also going to end shortly. She summarized her therapy thus:

Ms. C. M.: I've changed my whole attitude towards my ma. I've become cold with her. I'll do it when I'm ready to do it. I shut off something inside of me. My whole life used to revolve around whether mother was mad or not. I don't give a shit anymore. I'm also very well adjusted to the chemotherapy. As far as my scar goes, I look at the bare skin and I say I don't have cancer anymore so what the hell. I'll never say it looks nice.

Therapist: Good for you.

Ms. C. M.: I'm less and less with her. I've got to do it all myself and I'm going to. Now that I'm feeling more myself, I'm going to.

In sum, the patient was able, through the supportive therapy, to regain her self of vigor, always involved with fighting it out (and never leaving the fight) with her mother through eternity. The therapist's mirroring and idealized parental functions were instrumental in: 1) admiring and approving and giving value to her enfeebled self; 2) "taking over" the idealized parent functions of advising her and making policy temporarily.

This psychotherapy illustrates those situations in which the goal of supportive therapy was realized—equilibrium was restored—but the uniqueness of the patient's object world or selfobject world continued. Ms. C. M. and her mother continued to live in what we would call an archaic world.

CASE 2

Ms. J. K., a 26-year-old woman, came to psychotherapy seeking relief for her depression. She had become blind during the past year, a consequence of her diabetes. She had also been the recipient of a kidney one year previously which was now failing. In addition to these tragic events, she told of her mother's death from a stroke which happened directly after the onset of her blindness. Finally, her oldest brother, who had also been a diabetic and blind, had died four years previously, probably in a hypoglycemic state. Ms. J. K.'s psychological symptoms were that she experienced painful states of worthlessness and prolonged periods of crying and immobilization. Her environment was not helpful to her. Her surviving brother and father left her much of the day, so she relied on girlfriends to help her through the week. Even with the depressive symptoms, she was remarkably self-reliant. In her background information, she told of being the only girl in a family dominated by a tyrannical construction worker father and two older brothers. Her mother and she were the "hired help," depended on for the meals and the upkeep of the establishment. The patient described her mother as a depreciated person who stayed out of the way of her male progeny and husband. From early on her mother and she became, in effect, sisters in all respects and worked and played together in the service of the men. Although Ms. J. K. was an attractive person and had a lively intelligence when not emotionally retarded, the mirroring she received from childhood on was based on her Cinderella status in relation to her brothers and father and, later on, her mother. As she became older, her status with her mother changed and she went from a twinship relationship to one in which she became the protector of her mother against the verbal and physical abuses of her father and brothers. Her rages against the tyranny at home found another expression in her rebellious behavior at high school against the teachers and the system in her religiously dominated school. She tried to leave home at 18 and succeeded in staying away for nine months only to return again to the status of the surly female servant, thus joining her mother once more.

When her mother died, the patient's reaction was one of shock, not grief. There had already been quite enough in the way of separations, beginning with her brother's death, followed by her own kidney failure and blindness.

Ms. J. K. came to therapy because she could not tolerate the feeling of helplessness which she experienced; this was not as an ordinary accompaniment of the blindness but as inferiority, a manifestation of her ineptitude. The empathic diagnosis was clear, as was the therapeutic diagnosis. The patient was suffering with a self-collapse in which her experience of herself was that she was only a liability to one and all. Her endogenous sources of self-value were at a low level and her environment was seemingly without supports. The therapeutic diagnosis was that the psychic crisis demanded an infusion of mirroring and soothing direction-giving in a supportive psychotherapy.

The psychotherapy took place in two distinct phases: one in which the patient and therapist worked together in an attempt to form a self/selfobject bond which was relieving of her symptoms, followed by the second and last phase in which her condition massively deteriorated and the therapy was episodic, dominated by the therapist's attempts to comfort a hopelessly ill patient.

Phase 1a: The Formation of Rapport

The initial phase began with the patient's despair over her *abandonment*, in her view, by her family—by which she meant her brother and her father. They spent too little time with her; at times they did not even bother to call. She recalled many instances when she was alone in the hospital and no one in her family called for days. Her surviving brother and his wife, although they lived a short distance from her house, never called. Her father was away working or visiting with his drinking companions. Although she told of her mother's own failing condition—repeated strokes—coinciding with her failing eyesight and her final cerebrovascular accident, the patient did not allude to her mother leaving her until several months had passed in the therapy. The initial material sounded like this vignette, which was paradigmatic of the initial phase of relating and revealing her despair through complaints but rarely through direct expression of want.

Ms. J. K.: Everyone promises to call and drop in but no one stops. I told them, I told them. They all said they know I shouldn't be alone. My grandparents are fine. I said, "What am I doing? What am I doing that's wrong?" My brother works but gee-whiz, you get a lunch break, you can call sometime.

Therapist: Yes, I agree with you. I couldn't agree with you more.

Ms. J. K.: In the hospital this past Christmas no one in my family called me. I didn't get a call. My friends were fine. And New Year's on the transplant floor, no one. My aunt—just delivered a baby—she called. I was so angry. My brother and his wife they later said, "We're jerks." It's like beating a dead horse.

Therapist: That's just dreadful.

Ms. J. K.: My mom and I were close. Surrounded by boys, we were close. My dad is just *not* a home person. He goes out and does landscaping at other people's houses when he has free time. I guess when my blindness started, it was too much for her to take. She passed away just as my kidney failed. Tomorrow will be the first anniversary of her death. And who will remember her? No one. My grandma will. My brother won't remember. My father will remember but will not say anything.

Therapist: Your loneliness needs relief from people's voices.

Ms. J. K.: There isn't one steady piece of anything, no steady person.

Phase 1b: The Establishment of the Self/Selfobject Bond

The initial phase from the therapist's point of view involved the challenge of *posturing* himself to bring to this over-traumatized person a sense of worth that would diminish her pain. The therapist's task is made more difficult in these situations since there is always a great deal of the *therapist's transference* that has to be recognized and mastered. In this therapy, the therapist had to recognize from the beginning, and as it continued, the transference reaction of awe and futility, which was partially evoked by the patient's difficulty but was also well known to the therapist as the therapist's familiar inner experience when working with hopelessly ill patients (see remarks in Chapter 7).

Now the therapist's tasks—the supportive psychotherapist performing selfobject functions—are to offer at times the solace of the mirroring selfobject expressing *admiration,* while at the same time being able to demonstrate interest in the patient through clarifying-echoing responses. At other times in the same session, the supportive therapist will be the calmer-soother-guide, the functions of the idealized parent. In the case of this patient, the therapy started with the first session, as the need for support was apparent.

These initial sessions, in which the patient dealt with need-relating by complaints rather than by direct expressions of need, were reacted to by the therapist as the patient's justifiable *needs*— she had a right to expect that her emptiness and loneliness should be filled up with human support. Another special feature of dealing with this patient is quickly appreciated when working with the blind: at first, there must be more verbal input than in the case of the sighted, since no nonverbal cues are present. Thus the therapist had to be prepared to reveal to the patient that he was in touch with the patient's material by recasting or rephrasing or repeating.

Therapist: Must be hard to wait and wait now. Perhaps the hardest thing for you to get used to now is to wait for someone to do for you.

Ms. J. K.: Yeah, I'm not used to it. I don't want to be seen or treated like the kid. People don't understand; they call and say I'll see you, but then zero! I wait and wait and get lonelier and wow! What have I done wrong again! I can't just get in the car and see them. And then I can't shop at the store or make dinner . . . endless, endless!

Therapist: That's very understandable that you've got to have people plug into you.

This acknowledgment of the validity of her needs, in tandem with the actual expression of her needs, constituted the work of the supportive therapy for this patient: the combination of the calming-soothing aspects of the therapist's posture as well as the validation (mirroring) of the genuineness of her difficulties.

One other facet of the patient's self was in evidence early in the therapy: her defense against establishing a selfobject bond of nurturance. This is evident in the following excerpt:

Therapist: You're uneasy about people doing for you, aren't you? You weren't trained like that.

Ms. J. K.: I do feel uneasy. I want to do by myself. It's a hard thing to get used to. I don't want people to feel responsible for me. Like I'm some little kid or something.

In supportive psychotherapy this seeming paradox—the patient who is narcissistically depleted but resistive to the selfobject refueling—cannot be addressed or alleviated by a complete analysis of the fear of receptivity, but rather by the therapist acknowledging (tacitly) and accepting the defense transference against the selfobject transference. Clearly in this case, the therapist was aware from the outset that the patient had serious uneasiness in expressing directly to her uninvolved brother and father that she could not be left alone, since this was tied up with her feelings of inferiority. It turned out that the patient had a lifelong pattern of disappointment in the self/selfobject dyad of the self to be nurtured. Thus her complaints of loneliness and the delinquent selfobjects represented her way of defending herself against *her* incapacity to "be" the needy self and so be forced to put it into action. Thus, she could not do without the painful experience of ineptitude, the revived experience of the self being devalued and depreciated; her association with need was not one of joy but of inferiority. She could complain of the delinquency of her caretakers but simply not express her justifiable wants for safety or help. The therapist's mission became that of functioning as a selfobject who supplies the ingredients necessary for self-survival. In this case, the therapist had to continue his mirroring activities in as unobtrusive a manner as possible.

This initial period ended when the patient began to experience a decrease in her symptoms of despair and loneliness and became more vigorous. She entered a residential rehabilitation institute for the blind, attempting to improve her communicative skills and enhance her mobilization. The therapist continued to see her during this period and she was clearly in equilibrium. However, an ominous note was entering her life as she began complaining of having low blood sugar from time to time. She was now on

3x/week dialysis, but her uremia continued as well as its impact on her bone marrow; she was beginning to be more and more needy of transfusions.

Phase 2: Deterioration

Now, the second phase of the therapy came about when the patient started to physically deteriorate. The patient's diabetes began to go out of control, affecting all of her systems approximately one year after she began her therapy. The *essential* aspect of this therapy, which became in a sense the therapy of the dying person, was that the therapist was called on to "be" more of a selfobject, in the way of performing mirroring and calming-soothing functions. The patient, of course, with increasing uremia and frequent episodes of hypoglycemia, was commonly filled with malaise and mental confusion and slowdown, so that her self became even more enervated. Characteristically, this resulted in an increased experience of worthlessness, defining the therapist's task to infuse the patient with expression of worth. The following excerpts are from this patient's final session of psychotherapy.

Ms. J. K.: (*Pale, slowed down*) When is it all going to end? I'm so tired and sick of being sick and it's not getting better. I don't want to wake up in the morning. Nothing's going to change. Nothing's any different. I don't know whether I'll be on the floor in some emergency room or hospital by the end of the day. And it's so hard on my father. He keeps saying, Why did this happen to him? What did he do? He thinks it's in his genes that this has happened to me.

The therapist's task is clear but there must be an intrapsychic "clearing of the decks" before action can proceed, since the therapist's experiences must be optimally free of transference or countertransference contamination. In this instance, the therapist's experience of being with the patient was intense. She had deteriorated quickly, so that she seemed suddenly without any of her previous capacities to fend for herself. This was also manifest in her grooming, in the pallor and facial edema, and in the mental slowdown. The therapist reexperienced the feelings familiar to him of dealing with the terminally ill: the futility experience and the experience of awe. These were important experiences to be mastered since this patient needed company of a special kind—a reassuring, admiring, and calming presence:

Ms. J. K.: I need to get back on peritoneal dialysis.

Therapist: You've always been so good at going through these procedures. You're an excellent patient; we've always admired your capacity to go through these procedures.

Ms. J. K.: Well, I want to survive. It's really hard on my father now. Last time I was in the hospital, I was finally close to him. But it's hard on him.

Therapist: Here you are so sick and still thinking of others. You've always been special in that department, always thinking of others.

Ms. J. K.: Well, doesn't everyone think of their loved ones? It doesn't matter how sick I am. I could always think of my loved ones.

Therapist: No, you're special Judy, you always are.

Ms. J. K.: (*silence*) I want to thank you for all your support. I know it's your job but I know you couldn't do it without caring. I know I can always count on you, even if everything falls down around me.

Ms. J. K. died two weeks after this last session.

CASE 3

Mr. M. S.* was a middle-sized mesomorphic man in his early fifties who was referred by his internist for treatment of his depression. The internist had tried for two months to help him with appropriate doses of a tricyclic antidepressant. As Mr. M. S. entered the room in a vigorous manner, he did not exhibit depres-

---

*See Chapter 1, pp. 9–23, for initial data gathering.

siveness either in gait or overall appearance. He was neatly dressed but without a tie; the collar of his shirt was over his sport coat lapel; he was smiling.

He started outlining difficulties, which were that he had suffered a heart attack followed by a depressive reaction. He complained of feeling inept and useless and had lost the desire to go on living. In this initial interview he described some aspects of his premorbid self, especially his striving to be autonomous and unemotional.

The patient was revealed to be in a state of self-depletion, seemingly devoid of value of himself. As he pointed out, his self-collapse came about directly after his physical collapse, his heart attack. As he indicated in this initial interview (see Chapter 1) he had always identified himself as a self-reliant person; these traits had been challenged since his heart attack. In subsequent interviews he detailed the particulars of his early life which was filled with poverty, both materially and psychologically. He was one of eight children, the next to the youngest, and lived in squalor during his childhood and adolescence until he left home to enter the military. He remembered his early days with an admixture of grief and anger centered on the bleakness of his family life and the absence of positive responses to his needs. His mother, a harassed and depressed woman, seemed to him to be in a constant state of agitation but never was involved with him in an exclusive manner. He recalled no instances of physical or social intimacy from either of his parents. His father, an Orthodox Jew, was busy with either of his two major activities—junk peddling and prayer in the synagogue. He had always been a poor provider and each person in the family was forced to earn money almost as soon as he or she could read and write.

From an early age the patient would work with his father on the horse-driven wagon through the alleys of the west side of Chicago. Starting at eight years of age, he became successively a delivery boy (flowers, bakery goods), a janitor's helper, a maintenance man, a factory worker, and finally a taxi driver, until he entered the army at age 21. When he left his family to enter military service, he vowed never to return to a life of poverty.

After five years in the service as a signal corps specialist he returned to Chicago. He had effectively turned his back on his family by not communicating with any of his family. He learned that his father had died while he was overseas but he had not responded to any member of his family after receiving this information. When he returned to Chicago, he did inquire of a cousin about the circumstances of the surviving members of his family; however, he never returned to them.

He began work at a cleaning and dying plant and there met his future wife, another plant employee. Their relationship was, from the first, marked by a quiet mutual accommodation to each other's need for isolation. He soon became known for his hard work and he was quickly promoted finally to the position of the chief spotter in the cleaning plant. His industriousness extended into his personal life where he was always at work at some task around the house. Characteristically, he had little to do with the childrearing of their two daughters. He attended what various school functions he had to. Other aspects of his personal life were bleak. Apart from his work at the plant and his various chores around the house he did not engage in hobbies or athletics. His only nonwork activity was reading popular magazines, *Reader's Digest* or *Newsweek*.

When his therapy started, he was in a clear state of psychological disequilibrium. The empathic diagnosis was that he was suffering with an intense loss of self-worth which demanded immediate steps to effect a self-repair.

The therapeutic diagnosis was that he would derive benefit from supportive psychotherapy where the therapist had to *be* the idealized parent to offer succor to his enfeebled self.

The Course of the Psychotherapy

The empathic diagnosis for Mr. M. S. was that he was suffering a massive enfeeblement of his self so that he experienced himself as having little worth. He also suffered other vegetative signs of depression, including anorexia, malaise, and sleep disturbances. The precipitant for this self-collapse was the heart attack, which assaulted and defeated his only mode of receiving mirroring, his hypertrophied assertiveness. As soon as he realized he had to be quiescent for a relatively long spell, he reexperienced the depreciation that had always been associated in his mind with dependency.

The therapeutic diagnosis for this man who was immersed in a sheltered self was that he required supportive psychotherapy in an attempt to form a self/selfobject bond which, as we have previously noted, would hopefully alleviate the painful state of aloneness and diminished worth. During these states of self-collapse, many of the complex functions of the self—including self-observing functions, reality testing, and short-term memory—are not in operation or are not operating well. These findings alone would preclude the use of uncovering psychotherapy. Here we are citing these findings to make our therapeutic assignment clear: the patient's self is not in a cohesive state and requires the sustenance of supportive psychotherapy.

Phase 1: The Formation of Rapport

Mr. M. S. began his two-times-a-week therapy in the manner in which he began his initial diagnostic sessions, by complaining of his "laziness": "I just sit . . . sometimes for hours." These complaints would change to deriding complaints of his " . . . just feeling sorry for myself." During this first month of therapy, he railed at himself for a variety of errors and the use of poor judgment he had made throughout the years, ranging from marrying the "wrong" type of person to his allegedly poor performance at work. He also criticized his lack of humanism in general, and his poor performance as husband and father in particular.

The therapeutic task in this first phase was to provide a responsiveness that would be in harmony with his need to have relief from his aloneness, while at the same time not evoking any pain that would emerge in his self—through premature or tactless expressions of excess concern or warmth. The patient who is immersed in the experience of an enfeebled self, a self filled with hatred, responds to compliments with understandable rage since they represent a total lack of empathy and therefore a lack of compassion for the self-suffering with a profound loss of self-worth. In general, the therapist must be mindful in working with those patients who have received little positive mirroring in their life course to be cautious in dispensing admiring and approving comments. The reactions of such patients vary from the anxiety designated as the "flooding" response to mini-fragmentations with the lack of self-cohesion that emerges in these self-states where these is a temporary loss of self-esteem. All these reactions indicate that these patients still anticipate negative or painful responses to their self-needs for mirroring; therefore, any stimulation of these self-needs through compliments or warmth evokes the transference experiences of painful repudiation of these wants and ushers in the archaic fears.

The therapist's responses to Mr. M. S.'s complaints about himself in the first phase mainly consisted of being unqualifiedly accepting of his self-decisions. At the same time the therapist began little-by-little to insert comments—perhaps one or two in any session—pertaining to aspects of the interview material which revealed some positive aspects of his life in the past or in the present. These comments and the therapist's responses in general had to be expressed quietly so as not to tactlessly push the patient onto center stage and again be unempathic and therefore disrespectful of his experience of inferiority and inability to perform in any role at this moment.

A segment from this initial phase reveals this process:

Mr. M. S.: Well, I don't know why I'm here today. I'm certainly not going to be any different after this session. What could possibly change me? Any damn fool knows when a person screws up the way I did all these years. I don't know why they kept me all that time. All those garments I ruined. Yeah, well, I'll admit I did some things OK but I never showed the stuff that really good spotters show. And what about my life at home? What an excuse for a father I was! Did I ever take them out to a ballgame like other fathers? Did I ever take them out to a picnic? Or summer vacation? Or teach them hobbies?

And so now I sit. (*long pause, perhaps two minutes*) Lots of times there's nothing in my thoughts. Sometimes I have these nervous thoughts about the future and the present. Sometimes I pace, sometimes I sleep. I hate what I'm doing now—selling these greeting cards—but it's really no different than anything I'd be doing now.

Maybe all of you should just walk away from me. (*long pause, perhaps one minute*)

Therapist: It's a hard time when you're so filled with these negative feelings. They get so strong so that there's little else in your mind but these negative thoughts.

Mr. M. S.: I don't know about that. I think it's not just feelings. I have a pretty sad record of stupidity after stupidity. I just want to be left alone or put out of my misery. I wish everyone would just go away. Who's asking for all this sympathy? Actually my people keep looking at me like I'm some kind of freak, expecting me to just wake up and start behaving again. I'm not asking for anythin'. Why don't they leave me alone? (*pause, one minute*) I'm not askin' for much. Jesus, I've been keepin' food on the table for over 30 years. I just want to be left alone without their goddamn eyes on me all the time. (*pause, one minute*)

Therapist: You certainly have been able to provide well for your family all these years.

Mr. M. S.: I don't know. I guess so. She at least didn't have to work. But, what the hell good did it do? Here I am, I don't give a damn about nothing or nobody. No appetite for nothin'. Don't ever read the newspapers, don't even care who's in the newspapers. Sometimes I don't know what day of the week it is. I'd be better off 10 feet under.

But indeed, he did keep coming for therapy and missed very few sessions. Apart from the support in the sessions, the therapist gradually encouraged him to keep his business and to work at it as much as he could. The therapist met with his wife to explain to her that this phase of the depression would continue for some time and that her role in accepting his withdrawal and negativism was crucial. The therapist gave the patient and his wife some direction at this point, such as getting up as quickly as possible in the morning and engaging in some exercise like walking. Further, the therapist pointed out that it would be helpful to have an afternoon break for a nap. The therapist also instructed him in the use of certain ritual activities before going to sleep, such as taking a warm bath followed by reading to the accompaniment of special music.

Phase 2: The Establishment of the Self/Selfobject Bond

The essence of supportive psychotherapy lies in the establishment of the therapeutic bond which is, in fact, the establishment of a self/selfobject bond. This therapeutic bond in one sense represents the patient's unfolding needs to invest the therapist with features of the patient's original selfobjects. The transference that unfolds invests the therapist with either mirroring, idealizing, or twinship functions reflecting the patient's needs at these times. As we have stressed, the therapist in supportive therapy is called on to "be" the selfobject in his functioning as a therapeutic agent. The therapeutic diagnosis includes not only the diagnosis of what type of psychotherapy is indicated, but also the diagnosis of the nature of the unfolding selfobject transference and therefore directs the therapist to the indicated therapeutic posture. Although this posture may temporarily change from one session to another and sometimes within a session, it does maintain its centrality throughout the therapy.

In the first four-to-six weeks after the therapy began, the patient continued to fill the sessions with complaints about his inadequacies and occasionally about those of his environment, which included his "lousy business" and his unempathic (in his view) relatives. The therapeutic contributions were, as pointed out previously, to accept this outpouring of self-hatred without challenge and occasionally to offer a comment indicating a subdued appreciation of his circumstances and his background.

After this initial period, the patient began—little by little—to include the therapist in his inner world. He would say:

I felt like staying in bed today, turning my face to the wall and calling it a day or a life. Who cares about getting up, getting out, as you say? I certainly didn't feel like coming here. What's the sense of dragging you down with me? I could also hear you saying to me: "Get up, get out, it's going to make you feel worse if you don't move out in the morning." I got to admit I'm feeling less goofy since I've been here. Oh shit! So much crap in my life. A life of stupidity. . . .

At this point in the therapy, the patient developed a severe pain in his left shoulder, which radiated locally, and he was admitted to a nearby hospital for observation in the cardiac care unit. After being informed of this by Mr. M. S.'s wife, the therapist was able to visit with him the following day. The patient was then able to relate his fears about the possibility of another infarct and for the first time in the therapy he cried at the prospect of another hospitalization. He was also able to state that he appreciated the therapist's visit. The initial ECG did not show any new findings and that afternoon the laboratory reported that there had been no elevation of the pathognomonic enzymes, indicating there was no cardiac muscle injury. He did have a case of bursitis and arthritis of the shoulder joint and was sent home after two days.

When the therapist saw him later that week, Mr. M. S. reported again that he was frightened that his life was now to be that of the cardiac invalid and how sad this would be. Again he cried and associated to the sequelae of his childhood, especially the interpersonal aloneness. This session had little self-demeaning and criticism but rather was a session of mourning, a catharsis of grief in which the patient was able to ventilate the sadness of the past to feel sorrow for the deprived and frightened youngster he had been and who had been so precipitously evoked by the evidence of his illness and its forced dependency.

In the following weeks the sessions alternated between times filled with the usual complaining over his inadequacies and the new agenda: going over in some detail his work as the head spotter in the cleaning plant he had worked at for years prior to his myocardial infarct. The therapist's activity consisted of being the appreciator of his years of toil and creativity through appropriate comments. After this period the patient began to inquire what the therapist's thoughts were about his returning to the work of spotting. The therapist had known from other conversations with him and his internist that his cardiac status was in equilibrium. Further, the work of the spotter did not require strain that would be beyond his capacities. After inquiring about the extent of the duties, including the interpersonal encounters, and bearing in mind the patient's sensitivities over status as well, the therapist told him that resuming his activities as a spotter would be beneficial to his mental state. The therapist pointed out, of course, that he should check out with his internist as to the exact nature of the work so that he could go to his duties without any physiological anxiety. After a few more weeks of exploring the therapist's attitudes and his internist's comments, Mr. M. S. did start back at the cleaning plant three times a week.

After a few more weeks (six more sessions) Mr. M. S. decided that he would resume full-time duties as a spotter. He would not be the chief spotter, but the man who would be his chief was quite respectful of his wisdom; thus he felt without shame in working under him.

Phase 3: Termination

In the final two weeks prior to his going back to work full-time, there were some episodes of the old complaining and sadness but the major thrust of his sessions was going over in detail the follies of the world around him, at work and at home. He had disposed of the small business he had founded after his heart attack and was looking forward to a resumption of his old life, although he could not be the "jack-of-all-trades" that he had formerly been.

It was also clear that the old relationship he had developed with the therapist was now rapidly diminishing as he once again donned his character armor of being the hard-nosed compulsive character who depended on no one. The therapist was now observing the patient's premorbid self, replete with his put-downs of various groups of people, especially physicians! In the final interview, he began by complaining of the time it took to come to the office and the time it took for the psychotherapy session. Next he pointed out that the therapist looked tired and should be out of doors more frequently. As he looked around the office, he fastened on the microphone and commented that he would have a difficult time going over all the tapes that "we" made. He did not want to hear how he had sounded in the early stages of the therapy, because he was sure it was awful. Then, with a chuckle, he related how his work habits had returned to their previous form. He couldn't understand how people worked with such little zest.

For the rest of this final session, he went over with eagerness his work and his work habits. He felt he could now take over his "case," as he called it. Finally, he said that the therapist was "nice" in staying with him throughout his "weakness" as he called it. He was sure he was finished.

This was the last time therapist and patient saw each other. The patient did indeed go back to being a full-time spotter. One year later, the therapist heard from his wife that he had resumed the duties of a chief spotter and was well. The therapist has not heard from him or his family since that time.

In the next two chapters we will consider the psychotherapies needed for patients who are not in crisis. These are the clinical situations that require psychoanalytic psychotherapy or psychoanalysis.

5

Psychoanalytic Psychotherapy

The goal of intensive psychotherapy is to gain mastery over a self-deficit or to master through insight the fixations on archaic self/selfobject bonds. As previously described, patients requiring psychoanalytic, or intensive, psychotherapy are those with problems-in-living, where a major emphasis on the patient-to-therapist transference is not required or is contraindicated. These patients do not have those pervasive self or characterological problems that ordinarily require transference analysis for relief. The methodology of intensive psychotherapy reflects the emphasis on patients' problems in their environment. The overall approach is that the patient and therapist ally themselves to study the problem "out there," i.e., between the patient and the environmental situation that is evoking the self-distress.

THE COURSE OF PSYCHOTHERAPY

Once the empathic and therapeutic diagnoses are completed, the beginning stages of psychoanalytic psychotherapy focus on the establishment of an ambience of emotional safety based on the repeated experiences of uncritical acceptance of the patient and the content of his or her distress. Concurrently, the therapist begins his teaching assignment: the patient is to learn the techniques that will make him an ally, a partner of the therapist, in studying the conflict area that needs to be illuminated. One such basic technique or function is that of separating the self into the *observing* and *experiencing* parts, so that the patient begins the essential work of concentrating on his self-experiences in contrast to the emphasis on the outer world.

The therapist's first instructions to the patient in therapy are that the patient is to speak freely of his thoughts and feelings in the session and to focus on important events in his world. This is, in effect, a type of free association: the therapist tells the patient to speak freely but emphasizes that an important focus is on the environment in which the patient's problems have become manifest. The therapist's responses to the patient's material, especially in the early stages of therapy, set the tone for all subsequent sessions. The therapist will of course show interest via his facial and bodily tone but is to restrain his verbal responses so that the patient learns early in the therapeutic work that the patient will not be interrupted nor will he receive feedback after each association. The therapist stays away from "uh-huh" and "I see" and "of course" to each association and demonstrates this in the early sessions so that the patient becomes accustomed to the focus on his experiences rather than the instant feedback and mutuality that characterize conversation.

The therapist's affective responses, in the main nonverbal as we have indicated, are to reveal what is best described as "neutralized interest" (Basch, 1983b). The therapist is trying to convey as early as possible in the therapy that the sessions are in essence a laboratory in which two people are studying together; in this case the focus of the study is the inner world of the patient. The therapist's next task in the transformation of the patient into a research ally is to initiate the patient into the therapeutic alliance (Zetzel, 1956) or working alliance (Greenson, 1958). In order to do this, the therapist's instructions to the patient are that the patient and the therapist should now try to understand how the previous associations reflect a common theme or situation or distress. The therapist then recites the previous three, four, five, or six associations and in this way demonstrates the importance of following the associations and how they make up a universe of ideas and affects to be studied.

Another method of ushering in the mutual study is to announce to the patient that at this juncture "we" should take three steps back from this material and study it. The therapist then, as in the previous method, gathers the associations that together form an important message.

Another method is to say to the patient, "Let us draw a circle around this last material," or "Let us put this last sequence of associations under the microscope so we can study it." Again the therapist assembles the material, emphasizing the importance of following the connections and establishing the synthesis of the associations into an important universe of ideas and feelings. These directions have to be given repeatedly over many sessions in order for the patient to establish this process (Muslin et al., 1967).

Anticipating our later remarks on the curative factors in psychotherapy, we can say that after the patient gathers together his associations in alliance with the therapist, the work of tracing the material to its genetic roots can start so that the here-and-now concerns begin to reveal their archaic roots. After all, one of the basic missions of uncovering psychotherapy is to reveal over and over again the presence of the past in the present so that the reexperience of interacting and being gratified in an archaic self/ selfobject encounter is no longer possible without awareness.

CASE 1

Segments from the several stages of psychotherapy will now be presented. We will consider the psychotherapeutic course of Mr. L. B., whose diagnostic interview we studied previously (pp. 47–52).

Mr. L. B. is a 48-year-old man who presented himself for psychotherapy with the statement that his wife is threatening him with separation as a result of his distancing behavior in the marriage. He admitted to engaging in his sports and hobbies to the extent that it interfered with his marriage. After several sessions, it became clear that the patient's symptom of isolating himself from his wife represented a transference onto her from the patient's original caretaker. Further, the interviews revealed that his life is proceeding well in most other directions. The therapeutic diagnosis is that he requires understanding and mastery of this transference problem but he does not at this point require transference analysis to accomplish this goal.

Phase 1: The Entry into Psychotherapy

The initial task for the patient and therapist is to establish an ambience of safety in which the patient learns that unfolding of his self-issues evokes interest and attempts at understanding, not rebuff and misunderstanding. The next task is learning the basic rule of psychotherapy: the patient's task is to reveal all of his thoughts, feelings, and sensations, even as he experiences the intrapsychic pressure of shame, anxiety, or guilt dictating against disclosure. This basic and essential mode of communicating is to be entered into as best as the patient can, never to be compromised, even as the shame or other tensions become intense. On the therapist's side, his functioning is of course determined by his mission to gather the cognitive and empathic data, so that *abstinence,* as we have previously defined it (Chapter 1), is one of the cardinal features of the therapist's functioning, followed by the task (when indicated) of encouraging further unfolding of associated affective and cognitive material.

Now let us look at some vignettes of the initial sessions with Mr. L. B., which will demonstrate 1) the modes of communication of the patient that require instruction; 2) the therapist's attempt to elicit associated material; *and* 3) the therapist's attempt to encourage self-observing on the patient's part.

Therapist: Good to see you. Now that we're going to see each other two times a week, I want you to begin to speak freely of your activities during the week, remembering to be careful to say everything on your mind—thoughts, feelings, sensations—without restraint. If you and I watch it, the job of saying everything will become easier as we go along. I also want you to remember that at times I will not say much. I don't want to interfere with your thoughts.

Mr. L. B.: Well, I had a hard week. I told you a little about my son, Larry, and our car trouble. It's not the car, it's Larry and my wife against me on lots of issues. You know my wife *always* is right in her eyes. She *really* doesn't want me to shine, ever! Now this car crap. He's 25, about to get his MBA, and be off. He's a parasite, I pay for everything. Goddammit, I resent his taking my new car into all kinds of neighborhoods and parking it god knows where. She doesn't like me telling him to take the old station wagon and before I know it, the shit hits the fan and I'm getting it from all sides. If I kick him out, life will not be worth living with her.

Therapist: I guess you feel on the outside with them, unvalued.

Mr. L. B.: You said it. If she makes the rules, OK. If I say what should be, a war begins. In reality, the parking is bad around where he goes with his friends and I don't want my new car there. So what should I do?

Therapist: It's most important to get out in the open what you experience when you don't feel valued, like now with your wife and son over the handling of the car.

Mr. L. B.: You know these kind of scenes make me want to explode! I get a burning in my chest and I want to run. When she starts yelling that I'm wrong, I get mixed up and I lose my cool. It's like it discombobulates me. I don't know which way to turn then. I start to holler, I want to leave. Then I get angry at myself for being even less the general. When she opposes me and when they both oppose me, oh boy! I can't shrug it off then, it's no U.N. debate.

Therapist: This situation when significant people are not behind you is especially painful.

Mr. L. B.: (*long pause*) Many years ago in second grade—I guess I was seven—a girl snitched to the teacher that I was truant, that she had seen me playing around the house instead of going on to school. They of course went along with her charges. Whatever I said in my behalf was *nothing*. I had no mother or father to speak for *me*. (*pause*) No one is ever speaking in my behalf. I'm sure I never got invited to kids' houses or to parties because I had no mother. I was always different than the rest. (long pause) My aunt who raised me always left me out when she took her kids to the movies or for an outing. I was always the odd man out.

This vignette exemplifies the initial activities of the patient, after being given the necessary structure, in telling of his week with the experiences aroused by his interactions with his wife and son. Once the therapist had given the initial instructions of the basic rule and the focus on the events of the week, he then sat back to listen. He intervened to reflect back to the patient his empathic understanding of the material with an emphasis on the special experience the patient had described, a feeling of being unvalued. In relation to the patient's question, "What should I do?" the therapist now had the opportunity to teach another of the patient's tasks in therapy: to focus on his self-experiences, a psychological emphasis, rather than on the environment and its inhabitants, a sociological emphasis.

In sum, the therapist had now attempted to create the ambience of safety and had already revealed his basic posture of abstinence interrupted by his encouraging associated and affective expressions and self-observation (Wolf, 1976). He had also begun to isolate themes and issues with the patient, which would be continued and expanded in the next phase of the therapy.

Phase 2: The Therapeutic Alliance and the Problem-Centered Approach

The therapist's next task is to transform the patient into a work ally or a research ally since much of psychotherapy is a research project in which the research task is to uncover hidden influences on the patient's self-functioning. The therapeutic alliance or working alliance can be thought of as the transformation of the patient and his therapist into a work unit in which both participants are to study together the self of the patient. The therapist structures this alliance operationally, carves out of the patient's associations an important issue, a theme, a special self/selfobject situation, and then invites the patient to join in the study of this material.

Here is a segment from the fifth session with Mr. L. B.:

Mr. L. B.: Well, the weekend was fine. Last time we talked about my explosions. It sure would be nice if I didn't explode over everything and nothing. I lost some payment books for some real estate and before I knew it I was going to rip into everyone around me. I caught it and put it in place. Not everything is a big deal, not everything is a goof-up on my part, my badge of inferiority.

But I'm getting away from why I'm coming here, the separation stuff from my wife. She gave her OK to go ahead and buy the big TV. She's getting worried about you and me ganging up on her, like I'm getting more strength in here with you to defeat her and she doesn't want it. There are lots of things. She doesn't want to go to visit with my family, she says I get upset. She's wrong.

Well, what should I talk about today? I was kinda thinking today, what shall I talk about? Things are not going so badly.

Therapist: Let's go back now and put what you were associating about under the microscope: your inner experience that she doesn't want you to be strong tied up to her okaying the TV requisition.

In this instance, the therapist was putting together a critical pattern which had determined the patient's married life: his wife as the idealized selfobject transference figure who must, in his view, give her approval in all family matters. It is clear in this segment that this "complex" of transference was outside of his awareness, *not yet* a foreign object to be studied, a part of his self-functioning that he had, up to now, accepted. From this view, he was able to say without awareness: "Well, what should I talk about today?"

The patient ordinarily will not "get it" or "see it" the first time around, i.e., he will not immediately see that the therapist is uncovering a piece of his self that is important to be highlighted. In this case, what was illuminated was an archaic selfobject transference relationship in which Mr. L. B. was the subjugate, his wife the tyrant. We are coming up against the so-called *resistance* factor in psychotherapy, the patient's adhesiveness to ancient methods of maintaining intrapsychic peace. This resistance by definition obstructs the smooth unfolding of this or any therapy, so that the initial query cannot be addressed, the phenomenological "what." In this case, the "what" was the self/selfobject interaction that is being described. The second query of psychotherapy, "Where is *it* coming from?" will be answered out of the repeated associations to the theme isolated in the therapy, as will presently be demonstrated. It is important for the therapist to be mindful of the previous comments: The patient will not "get it" the first, second, or eleventh time, and so, for the reasons mentioned, the therapist repeats his confrontations, at times more directly, at times as a simple repetitious statement in harmony with the associations and always with the caution about overdoing a good thing.

Mr. L. B.: Well, she does want me to be tough at times. Like she certainly wants me to beat up on my nasty cousins and my aunt who raised me. Most people think I'm tough. At my office everyone thinks I'm a hard-ass. I'm not a wimp. I can talk to anyone even though I haven't had the breeding. I'm not into inferiority these days. I'm rambling I know. Maybe when I show intelligence, she doesn't like it.

What is clear in this brief segment (repeated several times) is that the patient is resisting the intrapsychic "what" and that the focus of the study is his self-*experience*, not his attempt to interpersonalize his situation and once again report on his wife's comments as if her directions are the sole determinant of his behavior. Mr. L. B.'s behavior will, the therapist surmised, be a reflection of *his* continuing striving to relive the self/selfobject fixation that has previously been uncovered. However, it is the patient's experience of his wife, of course, that determines his posture in *all* their interactions.

And so, the therapist, mindful of Freud's (1914) original admonition not to run away after the first comment regarding resistance is rejected, continued in his work to enlist the patient in an alliance of effort so that the work of self-observing the foreign body of the intruding self/selfobject experience could commence.

Therapist: Let's draw a circle around that comment, "She doesn't like it." That's the inner experience that's important, the sudden conviction that "she" is the authority, she is the boss, and it's nonnegotiable.

Mr. L. B.: Yeah, well, dammit she can do and say all kinds of things with all kinds of language and it's OK, but if I said what she says it'd be the start of another fight over my vulgarity. She can get away with all kinds of crap that I can't.

Here again the patient was insisting through his comments that "she" was the authority over whom he had no control. Directly after the therapist attempted to bring to his awareness that Mr. L. B. erected an image of a female goddess to whom he was subservient, the patient turned again to his apotheosis of his wife with his conviction that "she can get away with all kinds of crap. . . . " And once again the therapist had to wait without immediately engaging the patient in the alliance of mutual study. This resistance indicated that the self-split had not taken place: the patient was not yet able to study, to self-observe.

Later, in another session (#7), the therapist again was able to enlist the patient's self-observation in yet another attempt to encourage an alliance and thereby effect the self-split so that the study of the major interfering complex of Mr. L. B.'s life as outlined above could begin.

Mr. L. B.: We fight a lot over our son, the car and other nonsense but she always gets the last word, always the last shot. She has never agreed that I am right! Never, never, never, never! What can you do?

Therapist: Let's take three steps back from this experience that's common to you with her, that she's got the "word," that her words have the stamp of truth. What she values, you value.

Mr. L. B.: I do find that to be true. I gave in to her 100%. If she doesn't value it, I don't value it, whether it's a book or a movie. Boy, that is really something!

The therapist had to repeat many times the directions to gather together material and isolate it for observation and further associations in this early phase of therapy until the patient identified himself as the partner in the work and performed the required work without direction giving. Once this occurred, the therapeutic alliance was established.

The establishment of the alliance as described infers that a patient's self-observing functions have now become enhanced. This alliance is vulnerable to instances of regression, especially those situations in which the patient temporarily is in flight away from separation from his archaic selfobjects, i.e., fleeing from progress in the therapy. It is important to appreciate what the establishment of the alliance indicates to the self of the patient. The self of the patient has now been enabled to invest the self of the therapist with idealized and alter-ego selfobject features sufficient to allow the patient's self to experience the self-rewards of feeling calmed and soothed and invigorated in the presence of the therapist. A further gratification is experienced in the partnership of the mutual study aspect of the alliance, the revived feeling of the alter-ego twinship merger, the experience of "sameness," that special feeling of togetherness in the sharing of a project between an apprentice and his mentor.

In sum, this phase is ended when the patient has joined with the therapist in alliance behaviors *and* the patient and therapist have isolated a common theme or themes to study. It is important to repeat that this essential first step of therapy, the "what" of the distress almost always has to be outlined by the therapist. It is in essence a therapeutic confrontation.

Phase 3: The Working Through

Psychoanalytic psychotherapy has as a major goal the relief or mastery of a problem with which the patient is struggling "out there," i.e., in his environment. Psychoanalysis, on the other hand, is founded on the notion that when the patient intensely experiences the analyst as a revived significant parental figure involved in the patient's early difficulties, the patient can then review his ancient complaints, fears, and wishes of this figure and begin to grow away from the archaic objects with whom he is still merged. Psychotherapy cannot proceed without a special bond which must develop between the therapist and patient. This bond, the combination of the idealized transference (idealized parent imago transference) and the alter-ego twinship, goes into the establishment of the therapeutic alliance. The other experience derived from the psychotherapy transferences is that emanating specifically from the idealized parent imago transference, the calming-soothing direction-giving of this revived source of self-strength.

The psychotherapy proceeds with these selfobject bonds functioning silently for the most part, i.e., without the therapist attempting to highlight these transferences since the major focus of the treatment is on the difficulties with the figures in the patient's environment. Further on in this chapter, we will describe special situations in psychotherapy that do require the therapist to interpret the transference of the patient.

The working-through aspects of psychoanalytic psychotherapy, the so-called curative factors, begin after the patient and the therapist have identified a major "problem" of the patient, whether it be with a Ph.D. thesis that cannot be written or a love encounter that cannot be consummated. What does the working-through process in therapy entail? It is, in brief, the repetitious identifying and connecting the past with the present; it is the present dilemma being seen in connection with the past disappointments, fears, and rages that have made the self incompetent in these special situations.

To return to the particular therapy we are pursuing in this chapter, the self problem—the "what" of the therapy we have described—was that the patient was locked into structuring significant relationships, such as with his spouse, in repetition of the archaic and demeaning self/selfobject relationships of his past in which he became the subservient one and the significant other became the great disappointer. In this manner he continued, to relive his past in the present, frozen as it were in old, albeit painful, ties.

Psychotherapy of this type, we have said, rests on the establishment of an idealizing, alter-ego transference between the self of the patient and his experienced selfobject therapist. The patient and the therapist with whom he has established these therapeutic bonds now examine and uncover those situations in the patient's inner world that have interfered with his functioning in his current reality.

At times a special interference in the working-through becomes apparent at this stage or even earlier at the stage of the development of the therapeutic alliance: the intrusion of a defense transference. A defense transference represents the revival of a transference onto the therapist of attributes of a significant and depriving parental figure in one's development. The patient now reexperiences and reenacts the archaic manners of adjustment to this authority figure, whether it be compromise or subservience or decorativeness, in order to maintain the archaic self/selfobject equilibrium (see Chapter 2). In psychotherapy or psychoanalysis, the manifestation of the defense transference is a potent resistance against either the therapeutic selfobject transference (analysis) or the *therapeutic bond** necessary to examine the patient's environment (psychotherapy). In both analysis and therapy, the defense transference requires, at times, that the therapist or analyst interpret this transference so that the therapeutic bond or therapeutic transference can resume and therapy or analysis can proceed (Muslin, 1986).

During Mr. L. B.'s therapy, there were several instances in which the defense transference required interpretation. One such instance occurred in the third month of treatment when the therapist was delayed for several minutes in seeing the patient. The patient left the waiting room and went home. After 20 minutes he returned. This is the vignette:

---

*The transference of the patient onto his therapist is referred to as the "therapeutic bond" when it is not focused on or interpreted as it is in psychoanalysis proper. The therapeutic bond is a silent transference configuration of psychotherapy.

Mr. L. B.: I waited and you didn't come out and so I thought you were going to be busy and I left. Maybe I left too early but . . . I suppose that's why I came back.

Therapist: Well, let's try to understand. It was, after all, a matter of minutes.

Mr. L. B.: Well, at least 10.

Therapist: So let's get to work. What got stirred up sufficiently to make you get up and leave.

Mr. L. B.: My time is important, too. If you couldn't see me, OK, but waiting, that gets me uncorked. It's in the same category of being cheated, like with bills and that kind of thing. You know, people who are not really concerned whether you live or die, one number's as good as another for you. Like those untouchables in India, how do those people tolerate being treated like that? I have the same thing about concentration camps: how did those Jews let themselves be pushed into those camps and be killed? Nobody getting a gun and sticking it to them. Wow!

Boy, I'm getting far away from the thing we're talking about. Well, I admit it. I got pretty burned a little while ago but you know I must have been primed to explode like that and take off. I'm cooled off now, I guess. I knew I was making an ass of myself to take off like that.

Therapist: All these comments deal with being pushed around. And so, it was like me *making* you wait, like me the Nazi, you the concentration camp inmate without rights, stripped of all power.

Mr. L. B.: Yeah, well, you be careful of the time and I'll not run.

Therapist: It's a pattern that you find yourself slipping into: the other person becomes an unfeeling tyrant, you become the persecuted one. Today the old pattern came into this room. I became the tyrant, you came the victim.

Mr. L. B.: (*silence*) Yeah, well it wouldn't happen if you weren't late. (*silence*) I guess what you mean is some days I see putdowns all around me. That's true. Putdowns, putdowns. I grew up on them, never got the unconditional . . . the unconditional love people get when they have a mother.

Mr. L. B. (continued): Let me tell you what's been going on at home this week. . . .

The interpretations given dealt with the patient's attempt to transform the therapeutic relationship into one in which a reliving of the ancient mother (aunt)-son relationship would be effected, albeit one in which the patient had to reexperience the self-state of loneliness and inferiority which permeated his childhood. There were several other instances in the early and middle phases of the therapy where it became necessary for the therapist to interpret episodes of the defense transference impeding the major work of the psychotherapy, the illumination of the patient's difficulties with his milieu. In each instance, the patient experienced the action of the therapist as yet another manifestation of a lack of interest in his well-being. In each instance the therapist interpreted these reactions as reenactments of his defense transference now invading his therapeutic bond so that he was once again under the thumb or heel of the tyrant.

It is important to reemphasize that apart from these defense transference interpretations, there were no transference interpretations. Once the defense transference was diminished, the therapist did not respond to any transference manifestations.

The therapist and the patient whose treatment we are following now focused on understanding the problems the patient had brought to the therapy: his ungratifying relationship with his wife and others in his life. This working-through phase of the therapy, as we have described, consists of the repetitious tracing, and thereby illuminating of, the current malfunctioning relationship to those roots in the past that continue to infiltrate the present. In operation, the model of the therapy sessions can be charted in the following manner:

1) What is the patient experiencing? The operational aspect of this question, the phenomenological dimension, refers to the determination on the therapist's part to understand in detail the inner experience of the patient at any particular moment. Thus, when Mr. L. B. began the session describing a typical interaction with his wife that involved his provocative retreat from her followed by her anger, the therapist encouraged the patient to capture his inner world of experiences at the crucial juncture of his retreat. With the use of the therapeutic alliance and his selfobserving functions, the patient now would describe his inner world at that juncture with the admixture of affects and free associations sufficient for both therapist and patient to understand *what* was being experienced.

2) *Where is this reaction or experience coming from?* This is the second question in a psychotherapeutic inquiry. It refers to the genetic point of view and thereby illuminates the past-in-the-present aspect of the patient's experiences. Once again, after the therapist raises the question, the data are obtained from the patient's associations to an event or a special self/selfobject encounter, or the patient will draw a blank at that moment but will return to it later, or his next comment will offer a clue as to the genetics of his present behavior.

3) *What is this reaction or experience doing here now?* This is the inquiry that leads to the uncovering of the transference situation. After the *what* of the patient's experience is recognized and the background is uncovered, then the past-in-the-present can be more clearly illuminated as the *investment* in a current figure or situation can now be understood. The patient's past can now be observed living in his present relationship and, of course, interfering with his present relationships.

This scheme for understanding the data of a therapy session can at times be seen in pure form as it *spontaneously* emerges in a session. However, in practice the psychotherapist must be alert to maintaining a focus on the emerging material so as to *ensure* that there is attention paid to the phenomena of *what* is being experienced, *where* is it coming from, and *what* is "it" doing here *now?*

To resume our observations of Mr. L. B., we will now relate a vignette from a session in his working-through phase.

In this session, during the latter part of the first year of treatment, Mr. L. B. began by expressing his concern over his exhibiting to the therapist his successes as if he was always being a "hot dog." However, he said, he actually was doing quite well in his businesses and reeled off several successes over the past week. One success was in winning an argument with a female bank official over a loan previously denied him:

Mr. L. B.: She's not the type of woman who intimidates me, she's in her sixties, dumpy, and not sharp at all. Oh, I meant to tell you about my wife and her things with me this week. She and I have been fighting more. I guess I feel looser around her since my therapy started. I told her, you go see somebody if you feel so tense and argumentative. That must have gotten her shook, thinking I want to give *her* the heave-ho. She called me 10 minutes after that comment of mine. That's another vindication of me.

   She did something to me last week. My grandmother's sister and her husband are in town from California. My cousin called and invited us over. I said fine, but then the wife reminded me we have to go to an engagement party of a good friend's daughter. She said, if you want to visit them, you call up the friend and cancel. I'm not going to do that. She wouldn't let us go. She's tough.

Therapist: There's the old connection, the woman you experience as having power whom you *have* to kowtow to or else!

Mr. L. B.: You said a mouthful there! There are times when I'm with *that* woman I can't talk. I'm shaking inside and sometimes outside. Those people—they can be wearing pants—are so vicious, they got no feeling for people. One of the guys who works for me, he's always making jokes about cripples. He's always putting down people with disability, like he's bragging about his being a great jock. He needs to feel there's lots of people around him who are not up to him.

Therapist: You certainly are able to understand the problems that people with deficits have, especially their feelings of helplessness. With the tough woman you speak of, you *become* the helpless one. The woman you're with becomes the goddess.

Mr. L. B.: Why? Why do I become the punk? I have to remind myself with these people that I have the bucks, that I've achieved. I have the attacks, as I call them in the mornings. I shake all over. I feel like the little punk every morning. Is it because of the start I got in life? That was so long ago.

Therapist: When you're into these scenes with the powerful woman, before you know it you're lulled into that special experience of becoming the little one.

Mr. L. B.: Sometimes when I get disappointed if there's a chance of being disappointed, I'm kinda looking forward to it. I feel comfortable with things going wrong, or not being able to go or there's a very familiar ring. (*pause*)

Therapist: Sweet sorrow.

Mr. L. B.: Yeah. You can't go here because of this; someone failed me again! Sometimes, I feel good about it. Aha! You did it to me again! It isn't over! They're still doing it and I'm feeling good. It's so easy to figure out. That's what my childhood was which I didn't like then. I felt terrible. I remember walking by myself on summer days, nobody. Everybody is with their parents and I'm by myself and longing to have a family, to have a mother and a father, and it wasn't there.

Now, when I get disappointed, like my wife pulling this thing on Saturday night, I don't like it. At a different time it would have been perfect: Look what she's doing to me! It would have been perfect! *She's* not allowing me to show to my family. Now, I *don't* feel good about being disappointed. Before, I would have actually felt warm about it—isn't that the way it's supposed to be! Feeling good about being trampled on.

This vignette amplifies two of the three major queries:

1) "What" he was experiencing in those archaic self/selfobject relationships was the self of the youngster he used to be, the powerless "punk" at the mercy of the goddess. He also clarified a little later in the session that this powerlessness was associated with the feeling of pleasure associated with a promise of continui-

ty: " . . . it isn't over . . . they're still doing it to me." He related that disappointments and rebuffs evoked a familiar and pleasurable remembrance of the past old bonds, albeit with pain.

2) The second query, "Where does it come from?" dealt with the revived and relived archaic selfobject dyad requiring him to be in the posture of inferiority and resulted in him reminding himself of the painridden bonds of childhood. He recalled the sad longings and lookings for a parent who would embrace him and alleviate the painful aloneness.

The third query, "What is it doing here now?" could not be adequately illuminated in this session. As can be seen, the patient again demonstrated to us the pathogenic transference-in-action as he stated, "She's not allowing me to show to my family." This comment was a manifestation of his continuing transference onto his wife of those power traits he had always associated with the aunt who was his only parental figure. The vignette also demonstrated his diminutive self-experience in relation to this omnipotent figure: he could not go to the family as she did not give her consent. However, this material was not amplified in this session, although there had been much material uncovered about the self of the inept youngster who, while suffering so much in this sea of inferiority, *also* associated this self with the warmth of a bond, regardless of the associated pain of reexperiencing the self of the orphan. This genetic material is of course important in the reliving which the patient was undergoing with his wife, as the revived tyrant, the current "witch" who abused him. It is important to remember that the regulation of the work performed in psychotherapy is at the discretion of the therapist who must decide when there has been "enough" in the way of affects revealed, material uncovered, or interpretations which may cause self-flooding and a traumatic state. It is a common feature of psychotherapy that uncovering or working on significant material will spread over to and occupy several sessions; indeed, this work *requires* several sessions so that no traumatic self-flooding takes place.

The answer to the third query, "What is it doing here now?" referring to the malignant self/selfobject dyad which has been illuminated, *is* that the patient had been, up to now, fixated on only *one* selfobject whom he could trust as his source of stability (which he called "warmth"), although in order to maintain this dyad he had been in the self of servility. We can surmise that his parental figure only mirrored his self of inferiority and not much of it either. Thus, when he said, "She won't let me," he is, at that moment, totally unaware of his self-experience and what he had unconsciously made of his former peer, his wife.

Thus, this third query was addressed many times in the form of interpretations that Mr. L. B. experienced his wife as yet another version of his aunt which then "fixed" his posture. He would, the therapist said, then be compelled to wring his hands and complain loudly of the injustices meted out to him which he was powerless to modify:

Therapist: Here, once again, is that old experience now in relation to your wife where you protest that you're unable to influence her position. Like she's got the power, you're under her thumb. Once again we're looking at the old way of getting along with your aunt—it made complete sense, it seems to me, in those days for you to be passive with her, otherwise she'd leave you.

Mr. L. B.: Yeah, yeah. I always know how to get along with her. But with my wife, I don't know. I always argue with her. Maybe you're right. I always do feel she's got the smarts in the family.

Therapist: See, it seems to me that when you say "she's not letting me do this or that" you're into the old familiar experience of being with a tough, ungiving mother. And also you suddenly feel like you have no choice but to be on your knees or *else!*

Mr. L. B.: Yeah, but I know that she's not going to leave but do I really know that? I guess I do believe she's got the power, that's really nuts!

And now to the elaboration of the final inquiry: What is the phenomenon under our microscope—the archaic self/selfobject, as in this instance—doing here now or doing in this situation? We have uncovered that the patient experienced himself as a youngster in special situations, as for example with his wife, and experienced the other person as an idealized figure to whom he was subservient. Second, we have through his associations uncovered the data that are relevant to the question of where this phenomenon is coming from. The patient informed the therapist through his remembrances that being an inept, disappointed, and lonely person was associated with the warmth and togetherness—however minimal—of being "at home." The final inquiry deals with the question of what this aspect of the past is doing in the present, that is, what *function*, if any, is being served by this residue of the past. The understanding of this inquiry will bear directly on the central distress of this patient and his spouse. It will be recalled that Mr. L. B. entered therapy unable to devote himself to his wife, who complained bitterly of his inability to turn away from his sports activities to her.

Mr. L. B.: You know, she's a pistol. We were supposed to go out on the town Saturday night. Oh no! Her highness decides we're going to stay home with the tube. I wanted to go see a flick but all of a sudden we can't go! If *I* had decided to stay home and watch the tube, she would have had a fit. It's that way all the time, I never can say where we're going. She would just refuse and we wouldn't go anywhere. She's very stubborn. She always pulls that crap about how much better taste she has. Always rubs it in that I'm ill-bred, like I don't work. Shit! I'm getting more than a little pee-ohed at her snottiness.

Therapist: Well, let's try to understand. Sounds like we're looking again at you becoming the little guy looking up at a big shot.

Mr. L. B.: Yeah, I heard that as I was talkin'. We're still playing at the old stand. I certainly get into it a lot. It's not that I don't fight back. I've always fought back some, even with my aunt. She was always reminding me like my wife that I wasn't up to par or that my clothes were not right to go dancin' or some crap like that. She used to really hurt me when it came to that. She knew damn well that I couldn't dress better than I did. She took me for clothes like never and I couldn't make enough at those jobs for clothes I had in high school. Oh yeah, I used to fight with her but it was like fighting back. Actually I went along with her pretty near to 100%. She always had the last word.

Therapist: Well, here we are, the wife is experienced as a boss, like the boss you had in childhood. You suddenly experience her thoughts as coming from a goddess. The question is now that we understand these old ways of getting along in the past with the aunt, what are these experiences doing here now? What are these old patterns of getting along doing in your relationship with your wife? Once again the woman's comments are divine, never to be challenged. Once again you suddenly experience her as having absolute power and you have to go along with her.

Mr. L. B.: I don't know! I hate to suck around anyone. I never do it in my practice. You're right, you're right. Now what did you say, what are these old patterns doing in my marriage? What do I get out of it? Well, nothing—or less than nothing. But I'll tell you somethin', she sure as hell doesn't want me to be smart either! She's always putting down any opinion of mine, any magazine article I read. She says it's inferior. The name of the game is what do I get out of following her, putting her up there as you always tell me and putting me down.

Therapist: Yes, I suppose your wife does want to continue her leadership in the marriage as you've made it clear for many months, but it's your wishes also to *stay* under her that are now being revealed in your dealings with her.

Mr. L. B.: My wishes? I wish to stay in the hole, being pushed around. No! I'm not going to let her or anyone push me. It's true that it's kinda automatic for me to wait, you know, when I'm with gals. I wait for them to start talkin'.

Therapist: I think what I see as your wishes to stay "under" the woman are very understandable. It's really being in a relationship that's always been like home—you the little one, she the goddess. So long as you can stay being the little one and never show any longings to be assertive, to be tough, then you continue to be "safe."

Mr. L. B.: Safe, you mean safe like with my aunt, safe like she won't kick me out. Yeah, well I was very scared of that. God, I hate to be reminded of how scared I was of that little lady (*tearful*). How could people do that to a little kid? I sure took a lot of crap from that lady. I'll tell you a secret. These days when I come out of here and go home and we discuss something at home, I feel stronger. I know it's because you and I touched base, like a shot or somethin' like that. She don't like it when I'm smart, just like she don't like it because I'm a good father.

As can be seen from the last sentence, Mr. L. B. wished to continue to put his wife on a pedestal even as he was beginning to observe the transference displacement from the archaic selfobject aunt, the mother of his childhood. This last bit of transference intrusion—he the frightened youngster, she the purveyor of life and death—represented the work of the working-through process. And so the therapist and patient continued each session to dissect out of the patient's self-experience this limitation to his life: his diving into the archaic security of the self/selfobject dyad, based on his having to be inept, the other being the goddess. The therapist and patient would continue with the work until the endpoint had been reached, which would be evident when the patient announced that the symptoms of his experiencing himself as the inept one and the other as godlike were diminished or absent or much less troublesome. Here is an excerpt from a session three months later.

Mr. L. B.: You know, it's funny, I was home the other night and our son came in very late, half-crocked. "What crap is this?" I said to him, "You've got a big exam tomorrow night." I started to read the riot act to him but he was so crocked I sent him to bed. Then I went storming into her room, about to knock her down, to yell at her about the lousy job she did as he was growin' up. I usually tear him down, bawl her out. All of a sudden I stopped, son-of-a-gun, I was about to do it again. She's the boss and I'm about to complain, beat her down, beat him down. Goddammit, I'm the father, I'm the husband. I've been doing that all the time, like he and she are bosses, I'm the servant. I complain like hired help to the owners. I'm an owner! I bring home the bread and a lot of it, too!

You've been telling me for a long time how I become the "boarder," the poor visiting relative, in our house. But this was the first time I saw it with my own eyes. God, I hope it don't go away. I really saw it this time.

(Three months later)

Mr. L. B.: I believe I'm getting it under control. You know how I used to resist going one-on-one with our son, well I just realized I've been talking to him, just he and I, for a long time. I realized it because he and I were jawing the other night, probably pretty loud, and she jumped up and wanted in on the conversation. Well, I turned to her and gave her a mouthful about what we were arguing about and suddenly I burst out laughin' and I walked away. They were baffled like I wasn't playin' fair but I knew I had slipped, like an alcoholic.

(In a later session that week)

Mr. L. B.: I keep forgetting to tell you my wife has been going to the hockey games. Not all of them, but it's nicer when she goes. Also, I don't get so wild with her around, so it'll keep me alive a little longer! I still tape a lot of sports, though I don't watch so much as I used to. I really never had the time to watch all those tapes anyhow.

These vignettes are representative of the many instances of Mr. L. B. catching himself before becoming immersed into the transference onto his spouse and himself of the malignant archaic dyad of his childhood. The segments also demonstrate his increased involvement with the here-and-now aspects of his camaraderie with his wife and diminished dependence on the archaic bonds and archaic defenses of isolation. As the therapy progressed, one could see through these vignettes the increasing experience of the robust self, the enhancement of assertiveness.

At the end of the therapy, several self-transformations had taken place. Clearly, the patient now showed an enhanced capacity for self-observing. In line with this, his self-function of repression had become strengthened as archaic strivings appeared less and less. The pole of assertiveness as noted above was considerably strengthened as he now sought out people and activities in the here and now.

In summary, here are the self-changes that will have occurred at the end of uncovering psychotherapy:

1) The establishment of a therapeutic self/selfobject bond involving an alter-ego model (alliance) in combination with a mirroring (enhancement of self-vigor) selfobject bond and an idealized selfobject (direction giving and calming–soothing).
2) The development of insight into the original problem as it reveals the past in the present.
3) With the development of insight into past-in-the-present as it relates to the uncovering of archaic self/selfobject bonds, these strivings for the archaic mergers are considerably diminished.
4) The patient's self now experiences and strives for greater assertiveness. The pole of assertiveness can be said to be strengthened due to the establishment of the selfobject bonds, with an enhanced sense of well-being.
5) The patient's standards for himself have been raised.

These alterations in self-functioning *cannot* be said to represent more-or-less permanent self-transformations, i.e., self-changes due to the transmuting internalization seen in psychoanalysis proper, coming out of the optimal frustrations in a psychoanalysis. In psychoanalysis, the self-transformations are not strengthened *functions* as in psychotherapy, but represent *additions* through internalization of the selfobject functions of the analyst, and these can be said to be permanent additions to the self. After psychotherapy and the alleviation of a problem complex, the patient experiences a greater sense of well-being through the relief of the inhibitions due to the intrusion of an archaic complex. However, in a self psychology-oriented psychoanalysis, the endpoint of the analysis is the development of the self, the addition of internalizations from the selfobject functions to the patient's self.

Phase 4: The Termination

In psychoanalytic psychotherapy, the patient and therapist come to an agreement that the therapy can end. Almost always the patient initiates the termination when his or her symptoms are abated and the therapist agrees or expresses his or her concerns that more needs to be done. The therapist also has to be prepared to advise some patients who, while experiencing relief from their original problems, continue to have self-experiences that indicate a need for transference analysis, such as the pervasive experience of emptiness and aloneness or the sensitivity to rebuff followed by fragmentation experiences. These patients should be referred to psychoanalysis.

In psychoanalytic psychotherapy, the termination is ordinarily a matter of weeks as it does not involve the regression that is common in psychoanalytic termination. There is, on occasion, a temporary return of symptoms; and, of course, there are separation symptoms of anxiety and grief. However, these reactions lend themselves more or less readily to interpretation and support, dependent, of course, on the patient's sensitivities to separation (Goldberg, 1975; Palombo, 1982).

Mr. L. B. and his therapist agreed to a termination date which would come about in three months. The material in that period contained several sessions in which he remembered again instances in his past of forced aloneness which he had recounted in the therapy. He also remembered scenes of injustice with his aunt and mourned for himself as the deprived youngster who had suffered a great deal. On one of the weekends during the termination phase, Mr. L. B. had a return of one of his presenting symptoms. As in the old days, he turned back to his involvement with the sports on the television and walled himself off from interaction with his wife and family. He called the therapist on the Monday of that week and they had a special session filled with his complaints that he was "going nowhere, back to square one!" The next session found him again in equilibrium, reminding himself, without the therapist's interventions, that "that road was not going to be traveled anymore. I'm going to stay with people."

On another occasion towards the end of the three months' termination phase, Mr. L. B., with a very somber demeanor, started the session with a complaint that the therapist had shaved off several minutes of the previous session. He became morose and sadly commented that the therapist should know that these sessions were important and therefore be mindful of the time so as not to shorten the session. Fairness was a big thing to him and a psychotherapist, of all people, should know this. He became withdrawn for a considerable period of time and cried. The therapist had what turned out to be a final opportunity to interpret to him the defense transference, in which he experienced the therapist as the uncaring mother-figure to whom he had to beg for succor. After this session, the remaining sessions were filled with Mr. L. B.'s telling of plans for vacations and other leisure activities.

In the last session, he cried and told the therapist, "I want to know that I can call you when I'm in trouble." Mr. L. B. has not returned to therapy since termination several years ago, but he has called the therapist a few times to tell of his progress and his son's accomplishments.

CASE 2

We will now present the course of psychoanalytic psychotherapy for Ms. A. R., a 38-year-old housewife, referred by her internist for treatment of a phobia. For the past several months she had become increasingly frightened of leaving her home. She related that six months ago on the airplane returning from her parents' home in Tucson, Arizona, the frightening idea came into her mind that the plane would explode in mid-air or crash on landing. This trip was especially trying to her since she had been informed that her father was suffering from end-stage kidney illness, and now her parents would no longer be able to visit her in Chicago. The entire return trip was in her view "like coming back from a funeral." In her diagnostic interview she told of her childhood, which was marked by illness and separations from her family. She was told that she had been born with a congenital dislocation of her hip and apparently, after many consultations with physicians, the diagnosis was made that she would need hospitalization for a lengthy period to effect the correction. At age six she was again taken away from her family to a hospital for several weeks, this time for treatment of swollen joints as she had become ill with rheumatoid arthritis. These joint problems continued to plague her off and on until the third year of high school. Since that time, with only one short relapse for knee swelling, she has been in remission.

Equally as important in her history was the history of her self-experience throughout this childhood of pain and isolation. In her view Ms. A. R. never received the psychic nurturance she required as a youngster to overcome these repeated threats to union with her selfobjects. Her mother apparently became overwhelmed by her daughter's illness and often complained that she was a great burden to her, especially since she so frequently complained to her of her pains and distress and was unable to be calmed. On the contrary, she had difficulty in sleeping, was a bedwetter until she was eight, and was a binge eater throughout her childhood. She also had a great deal of fear attached to going to school and even going out to play after school.

Ms. A. R. also told in the diagnostic interviews of another recent family stress. A few years prior to her father's increasing difficulties, it had come to light that he was an addicted gambler who had squandered the family savings. It was a great shock to Ms. A. R. and her older brother (two years her senior) since their parents' marriage was always held out to them as a perfect union and her father was especially revered in their family. Since that time, her mother had become uncharacteristically dependent on her and her sister, calling each of them frequently and clearly investing them with parental powers to be her guide.

Another recent stress on Ms. A. R.'s self-cohesiveness had been the emergence of her husband's success as a corporate attorney which necessitated his being away from the family for increasingly long periods of time. They had a 12-year marriage, which until three-to-four years previously had been an important source of stability to her. They had entered into the parenting functions and community involvements with enthusiasm. He was always identified as the highly intelligent and achieving "brain" in the family, she as the pragmatic commander of the family ship. Although they apparently had little in the way of romantic love, they were devoted to each other and their children (two daughters). The patient experienced her spouse's now-frequent absences as a major loss to her sense of well-being, and she became refamiliarized with the feeling of isolation.

To complete the story of her development, the patient told of her years in school as being years of uneasiness until she learned to suppress her neediness and passivity. From her mother's emphasis on being decorative and accommodating to males, she became, in secondary school, determined to be "popular." She was able to suppress her overeating and introversion and thrust herself into groups and into the local social scene. When she went to college she was already an accomplished interactor and had many beaus. She became engaged to her husband in her last year of college and they married shortly after her graduation.

Returning to her major symptom, Ms. A. R. said that at the present time when she was to leave the house, she became aware of the experience of fear. She could not trace it to a specific happening, past, present or future, nor could she state what might be frightening to her in the trip or the specific location to which she was journeying. At times she would cry as she became distraught and would begin to rock herself to-and-fro. During these times she would call a friend, her sister, or her mother "just to hear a voice that will calm me."

The empathic diagnosis was that of a self in chaos evoked by a series of separations from selfobjects. The resulting self was becoming more and more enfeebled and needy of narcissistic supplies. From what we have observed, the patient had been harboring a fear of aloneness since being left alone as a youngster, suffering with the emotional vicissitudes of two major illnesses. Unfortunately, she had also learned early in her life that exposing one's longings and strivings and uneasiness to her caretakers would evoke abandonment or at least disdain.

The therapeutic diagnosis was that she would benefit most from a mixture of supportive and uncovering psychotherapy. At this point the patient was still somewhat in a state of self-disarray; she was not able to be adequately calmed. On the other hand, her disarray was circumscribed. She could identify her problem as being intrapsychic, yet she could not of course control her phobia. In many parts of her life she was in good equilibrium, and until her most recent trauma and subsequent disarray she was identified as a leader in her community. Thus she had an identifiable problem in a self that until now had been able to be cohesive and therefore did not require analysis. The therapeutic diagnosis of supportive and uncovering therapy was at this point predictive since there was little evidence to attest to the existence of a capacity for self-observing (and therefore the capacity for an alliance).

After the diagnostic period of six sessions, the therapist informed Ms. A. R. of his impressions of the indicated therapy and the times required. She agreed to coming in two times a week, and mutually acceptable times were arranged.

Phase 1: The Entry into Psychotherapy

The initial sessions were filled with the patient's *uneasiness* over being unable to fulfill social obligations which required travel out of the state or at great distances from her house. She became convinced that her forced passivity would evoke contempt and rejection from her family and friends; she erupted on several occasions with accusations against her husband that he was planning to leave her. Her husband became so distressed by this unusual behavior on the part of his wife that he called and arranged for an appointment with the therapist, which his wife heartily endorsed. She was very eager for the therapist to explain to him that she required him to be accommodating to her now. In the meeting with the husband it was clear that he had become dismayed by the transformation in his wife from a noncomplaining, ever-accepting person to someone who suddenly needed constant reminders that he was not angry with her and would not desert her in her time of need. At times she had become near-violent in her need for him to demonstrate his loyalty to her. The husband asked the therapist to see his wife more often, claiming that the pressure on him was overwhelming. He accepted the therapist's overview of her psychological situation and promised that from his side he would not be impatient for her to resume her social and business obligations.

The patient felt some relief from the therapist's meeting with her husband, but the tension continued. She revealed that she talked to her mother in Arizona daily but now the calls were filled with *her* crying since she found herself each day begging her mother to understand her plight. In association to this, she related the tale frequently told by her mother that she had always been a difficult child. Her mother told her repeatedly that she was a great burden to her, that she was so difficult to raise. The patient repeated to the therapist at this point the list of her childhood difficulties: bedwetting, overeating, nailbiting, clamoring for attention, school phobia, hyperkinetic behavior. She vaguely remembered her hospitalizations as fearful events. She was all alone in this foreboding place except for her father. Her mother did not visit her (later corroborated by her mother) since she was apparently too distraught over her daughter's illness. Some of her hospitalizations she remembered more positively; the physicians and nurses were helpful and supportive and she was helped in obtaining relief from pain.

She remembered that directly after the hospitalization for arthritis her behavior underwent a major shift, from clamoring to her mother for attention to total subservience to her mother's wishes. Her mother had preached to her from early on to concentrate on her grooming, her figure, and her dress so as to always present an attractive face to the world, especially men. She worked hard to become slim and gregarious so that when she entered high school she was "popular" with everyone, especially boys. The greatest transformation took place in her relationship with her mother as she now, in concert with her brother and father, gave mother center stage so as to allow her mother to continue to be the queen of the family. From then until now the patient had accepted the family code: in discussions with the mother, one is allowed a few short sentences centering on one's issues, then mother takes over in an atmosphere of obedience. The patient had discovered early in her life through the learning experience of being actually abandoned in hospitals that in order to have a mother who would be the figure responsible for her life, she must adopt the permanent posture of subservience. It is no wonder then that the patient cried daily to her mother (and in the past to the maternal surrogate, her husband) for understanding and commiseration. She was fearful that once again, whenever *she* expressed a need, she would be rebuffed and even abandoned.

Now in her therapy, she asked at each session about the feasibility of a tranquilizer or any other method that would speed up the therapy. She even questioned whether she could see a behavior therapist so as to speed up her progress. She cried over her inability to give up her phobias, again fearful that "people" would resent her infirmities, that no one would understand.

The therapist's activity during this initial phase was focused on establishing an ambience of safety, to function as the idealized parent who *had* to calm her. This selfobject function was accomplished in various ways, among them reminding her of her victimizations: she had through no fault of her own suffered serious illnesses in the past as in the present. Another calming function was to remind her of her husband's unswerving loyalty to her and to their family for 12 years.

This initial phase was ended when the patient entered into a therapeutic self/selfobject bond and could now experience the relief of the calming functions of the idealized bond. She could now without difficulty travel by herself several miles to her sessions. The daily sessions of clamoring for pity to her mother and maternal surrogates ceased. She had gone to the heart of the city, which was a considerable drive, a few times already, albeit with trepidation. The bonding had been achieved with no specific attention (such as interpretations) required to the defense transference in her psychotherapy since, although it was clear that she exhibited those features of this posture—the little, whining, pitiful person in a state of subservience to the vaunted authority figure from whom she hid longings and strivings—she responded to the therapeutic ministrations of support by entering into a therapeutic bond and felt uplifted. If the clamoring behavior to the therapist had continued without abatement and she continued interminably to feel painfully defective, the therapist would have been required, after "seeing" this defense transference posture, to neutralize her defensive posture and her transference through interpretations.

Phase 2: The Therapeutic Alliance and the Problem-Centered Approach

After the bond had been achieved, the therapy could now center on the self-injury which was evoked by the precipitant event: the fearful weakening of the archaic self/selfobject bond between the patient and her mother when the disease of her father permanently altered, in the patient's view, the relationship between herself and her mother. What had actually been altered? On the surface, little in reality was transformed, since for several years the mother had had little impact on the grown-up woman who ran her own family and was an effective figure in her social world and in her husband's business world. No, nothing had been altered to affect her present-day circumstances. What had been altered was that intrapsychic unconscious remembrances had been evoked: the archaic experiences of the defective childhood self abandoned in a hospital or in a physician's consulting room. Weakening the archaic self/selfobject bond would produce the fragmented state-of-self. Needing the balm of the idealized parent selfobject would reproduce the abandonment experiences of childhood since the selfobject in the patient's conviction would abandon her even further when she revealed her manifest self-needs, as she had so often done in the past with tragic consequences.

It may be of some interest to attempt to articulate the rationale or even the necessity for pursuing the issues of psychologically clarifying (i.e., explicating to the patient) the dynamic of her retained bonds to her mother and all the maternal clones to whom she had become attached through the years—husband, girlfriends, children. This patient had continued in her adult life, albeit unconsciously, to maintain the archaic bonds between her impaired self of childhood and the maternal selfobject. In many significant encounters in her present life, she slipped into these self-transformations in which the maternal selfobject or its clone became the apotheosized figure and she entered into the reflex subservience. In these encounters, as we have documented, she became stifled vis-à-vis her other more reality-oriented needs as she became frightened at the prospect of displeasing, which would result in abandonment and self-fragmentation. Therefore, the therapeutic task was for the patient to extricate herself from this unconscious imprisonment of the past and its archaic selfobject world and usher in the here-and-now self and the world of the present, where her needs for empathy and compassion would be recognized and hopefully gratified.

The therapeutic issues were clear: to attempt to focus with her on the *what* issue, the specific scene that had at its core the entry of her self into the malignant self/selfobject encounters where she was to be the defective self pleading for her psychic life, the other to be the queenly selfobject, the purveyor of her worth and even her mortal life. Several therapeutic encounters will now be described which will highlight these therapeutic movements.

The patient could readily recognize the fears she experienced on the return trip from Arizona which ushered in the phobia. The state of aloneness which she entered into was familiar to her and when the therapist pointed it out to her, she could "see" the phenomenon, the "what" of the situation, and begin to isolate it and hook it up to relevant remembrances of other times of aloneness. Here is an excerpt from the middle of the 18th session:

Ms. A. R.: I felt kind of in a fog today. It wasn't bad but it reminded me of the way I felt when I finally understood that Dad was never going to be the same. My mother was so upset and you know, I couldn't comfort her. I started going to pieces. Wow! (*cries with shaking sobs, long pause after crying*) I'm sorry, what can I say, I fell into little pieces.

Therapist: Well, let's now try to take three steps back and look together. Now that we've heard this special reaction you had several times, maybe we can try to put it under the microscope and study it better so we can understand what happened. It sounds like you actually *became* the frightened youngster, all alone without a leader, when mother became immersed in her distress.

Ms. A. R.: Yes. (*weeping softly*) I did, and yes, I do. It's so hard to contain myself each time she calls now, I go into the same routine. Alone you said? Maybe that's it. Alone. (*cries*) Maybe that's it. 'Course she's going to be alone. My dad is *not* going to recover. (*cries, long pause*) I'm going to have to go out there. Can I? Will I ever be able to fly again? Oh my, my mother all alone. (*pause*)

But you said I'm alone and I became the kid again. You meant when I was a kid and I wouldn't go to school and all that stuff and became a brat over and over again.

I'll tell you one thing. I certainly have had more crying spells since I've been home from Arizona. The other day, in a department store, the clerk had a little edge to her voice, you know what I mean? She didn't mean anything, probably tired. She just couldn't be pleasant counting up change and gave me a cold look. Wow! My heart sank to . . . to my ankles. I felt empty all over.

Therapist: Like you suddenly needed company, a leader, a strong right arm. All alone again.

Ms. A. R.: Oh yeah! All alone. (*cries*)

This type of scenario, repeated several times and in many different settings, helped usher in the awareness that Ms. A. R. was at this time in her life reactive to any *threats* to dissolution of interpersonal bonds, even the bonds of a slight contact made with a department store clerk. Each time she experienced an attack on any of her relationships through a complaint from mother, hus-

band, children, she experienced the familiar dread and took whatever steps were necessary to mitigate the complaint. With her
husband, she related:

> My husband came home very late last night and I had al-
> ready gone to sleep. I tried to stay up but I couldn't make it.
> This morning he was so surly at breakfast, you know what I
> mean? I said, OK, let's have it. He finally said something
> like, "You're trying to punish me, you're trying to punish
> me, why do you do that? You are punishing me! I come home
> after an exhausting trip. Where are you? What's the sense of
> me busting my ass out there to come home to nothing!" I
> tried to tell him I was exhausted after running the kids all
> around but all-of-a-sudden I said to myself, you know I think
> he's right. Maybe I am punishing him. I have been angry at
> him for years about this leaving me alone I told you about.

With a womanfriend, she related:

> I called up my friend Sue and told her we couldn't go to
> Florida with her and her family. I told her I was run down
> and my husband couldn't promise a date over the next few
> months because of some matter in his firm that needed him
> to be around. She was *so* disappointed. She reminded me
> that it was my idea and I had gotten her and her husband all
> excited about the idea and now I was letting them down.
> (*cries*) She said that I wasn't being fair. Well, I went nuts! I
> started to cry and begged her to forgive me but I just couldn't
> go now. She was so shook at my behavior that *she* began to
> cry and finally told me to calm down, she only meant she
> was disappointed.

In response to these associations to the threat of a rupture in
the relationship, the therapist again confronted the patient with
the self/selfobject situation in each of these encounters. He said:

> In these situations with your husband and with your friend,
> the "what" of the situation that we're looking at is again you

entering into the little person self, frightened that your leader is leaving your side, and so you rush to join his or her side by agreeing or apologizing so that no one leaves you. When your husband or friend is in a disagreement with you, there is *distance* between you and them. This distance frightens you. You quickly do whatever you have to do to cut down the distance—agree, apologize, or whatever is needed.

After many more associations revolving around the theme of the threatened self/selfobject bond, the patient and therapist were ready for the next therapeutic phase which centered on the illumination of the patient's background, the history of her relationships with significant figures. The therapeutic task was to render the "problem" therapist and patient were working on even more self-alien, always looking at it as an object for study.

Phase 3a: The Working Through (Initial Phase)

For learning and teaching purposes we are isolating the phase of uncovering the patient's background as if it always is to follow the previous stage in a lockstep manner. In practice, the query, "Where does *this* (interaction, sensitivity, role, defense) come from?" at times follows on the heels of the previous query, "What are we looking at here?" In other instances, the queries follow in one session or in one piece of material. However, it is heuristically useful to separate the query from the material that emanates from a study of the patient's history of relationships and history of self-fixations and self-transformations over time.

In this patient, the "where does it come from" query was initiated after sufficient illumination, in the therapist's judgment, of the problem sector: the continuing sensitivity over the *threat* to an interpersonal bond. Now the therapist said something along the lines of:

I think we're clear that you enter into this special experience. The other person—mother, husband, brother, friend—is suddenly dissatisfied or critical of you. You become uneasy, at times filled with dread. This dread mobilizes you into what-

ever action is required to bring that person around to find
you again an acceptable person. We've got to turn our attention at this time to where this complex of experiences comes
from, to what does this dread of abandonment hearken
back? I believe we are both convinced that you do not simply
fear rejection at this point by your friends or husband. The
dread is too strong. It's like you're reacting to an old movie
which at the moment of dread you are unaware of even
though it has crowded into your mind.

The above comment, of course, is an elaboration of the comment
that was actually made: "Where does this uneasiness come from?
This dread must have an antecedent somewhere in your background."

In response to this repeated query, the patient began to tell the
therapist in relation to the present fear that she had always "glori-
fied" her mother and her opinions and did not remember when
she had not been in contact with her at least one time a day,
including weekends, holidays, and even during her honeymoon.
However, in her childhood she remembered being left in hospitals
and not being able to see her mother. Each time she was taken to
the hospital it was by her father; she never remembered seeing
her mother during *any* of her hospitalizations. Although her
mother had often disagreed with her about this matter, the patient
always maintained that her mother *never* visited her during her
stays in the hospital for her hip difficulties and later for her joint
problems. She did not remember when her overeating began nor
her "disagreeable" behavior of whining and crabbiness, but it was
throughout her childhood. As she told it now, there began in her
childhood a sequence of behaviors that was often repeated: She
would initiate a discussion with her mother by complaining of
something that was disturbing her. These complaints were accompanied by tears and whining behaviors. Her mother would respond by becoming distressed and complain to her that she, our
patient, was a source of great difficulty to her, why couldn't she
pattern herself after her brother? The patient, in reaction to this
rejecting remark, became even more distressed. Her mother,

now markedly distressed, would leave whatever room she was in. Our patient would run after her. This scene apparently was repeated often. At times the father would enter the interaction, always on the side of the mother.

The therapist and patient never did uncover what combination of environmental influences and maternal rejections helped the patient in mid-high school to extricate herself from these scenes with her family, but she did become involved with boys, clothes, and parties somewhere around her 16th birthday. The daily mournful contact with her mother continued, as noted to this day, but in a diminished form. From mid-adolescence to the present episode of psychic disarray her external behaviors were marked by a gregariousness that was the converse of her childhood self of despair. Always on the go, always with a smile, she became the high school homecoming queen in her senior year and was voted the most popular girl in her school. Her inner experience during this time, and in the present as she related it, had always been marked by an awareness of anxiety in relationships if she disappointed, if the other person became dissatisfied or critical, or there was *any* sign of disagreement. In sum, the patient had effected a *self-repair* in adolescence in an attempt to overcome her fears of abandonment. This self-repair amounted to a self-split, the clamoring self of childhood walled off from the rest of her psyche, the more adult self, which became that of the effusive, service-oriented self. The needs for calming and approval of her self were now hidden from view (repressed, horizontally split-off) out of fear of abandonment should these needs again be exposed.

With repeated externalization of these instances of the patient's background of fears of rejection whenever was in a state of need, our query, "Where does this complex of fears and idealization and subservience come from?" was sufficiently answered.

Phase 3b: The Working Through (Final Phase)

This phase represents the work done when therapist and patient (alliance behaviors) center on the final therapeutic query: "What is the complex of subservience doing here now?" This query deals with the insight of the *past* in the *present*, the transference from the significant parent onto the current significant figure(s) and from the self of the patient in childhood onto the self of the patient in the present. The psychological importance of these resurrections, the unconscious importance of these intrapsychic relivings of the past, is, of course, idiosyncratic and therefore must be understood as having a unique purpose in each instance. In one instance, the therapeutic problem and its past-in-the-present process contains the self-need to reestablish the defense transference to capture again the archaic security, albeit by relinquishing in large part the mature self and its accomplishments. In another instance, the return of the archaic self/selfobject dyad is reinvoked or erupts from time to time in an attempt to evoke from the resurrected and elevated parent figure (the transference selfobject) the heretofore missing selfobject gratifications.

The query in operation is sometimes best articulated as a question, "What is it (the revealed complex) doing here now?" At other times the query is best articulated as an interpretation: "At this time you are on the one hand investing your spouse (friend, child) with the qualities of your father. On the other hand, you are diving into the self of childhood, again apologizing to your invested authority figure." This interpretation in this phase is a more complete version of the interpretation given to the patient in Phase 2 when the therapist can only say, "You become the youngster, he becomes the authority." In this phase, after illuminating the genetic background, the therapist can say, "On the one hand you elevate your spouse (brother, child) into the *role* of the Queen mother, the mother of your childhood. On the other hand, you dive into the self of childhood, the little kid who could only get along by being subservient."

How are these operations *curative* of the patient's distresses? Once the therapist begins to encourage the patient to achieve insight into the unconscious transferential aspect of his presenting problem, he has initiated the primary curative process of psychoanalytic psychotherapy: the patient and therapist in a state of alliance studying the data. Thus, for example, a patient, caught up in the repetitious need to form idealizing relationships in which he *always* becomes the vassal, stifling his wants for recognition and consequently suffering with lifelong emptiness, is in dire need of illuminating this anti-life repetitiousness which has thus far *inhibited* his longings for support. Once this investigation is launched in the therapy and the patient and therapist are joined in ferreting out from the patient's self this repetitive and destructive structuring of relationships, the self-observing *process* that is initiated continues to act in self-observing outside of the therapy session so that ultimately it (the self-observing function) becomes an effective restraint acting in opposition to the patient's previously unchallenged and automatic self-defeating urgings. We must add immediately, self-defeating to his 1987 aspirations not to his 1957 or 1947 aspirations, where the repetitious establishment of an archaic bond to petition for succor in the self mode of an unformed youngster was not out of tune and therefore not evocative of shame.

Segments from this phase of the psychotherapy in the case of Ms. A. R. follow:

Ms. A. R.: Crazy how I sometimes get into a snit with my husband and act so dumb and like a slave to all his thoughts. Like I suddenly don't know who the hell he is. I mean I love him but gee-whiz he's not the last word on everything. I can forget, just like that (*snaps fingers*) that he's been coming to me for years with all these questions about people and what to say, what to do, and so on. I know there's some connection between my mother's comings and goings. You know she just left. I guess this time in many ways was the worst visit— well, the worst and I suppose some progress as you would call it. She really does say mundane things and over and over and over. Wow, can she spin a web of importance over nothing. I swear if I hear that story again about *her* problems with *her* mother that'll be the end! If I hear those stories again about her being an expert wife and how I should do this and do that to my husband. Like my kids say, it sucks. That same old crap she fed me, all that shit about what you're supposed to look like, the woman never read a book in her life. And if you try to tell *her* something, anything new that she never heard of, she rushes to change the subject. Ah, listen to me, she's already an old lady. (*long pause; begins to quietly whimper; recovers*)

I suddenly started thinking about this crap with my husband. I'm embarrassed to tell you what we fought about. (*pause*) He wasn't fighting, I was. Over his pushing me—oh, goddammit, he wasn't pushing me. He just said, we have to talk about our daughter's new bike. The cost. I blew up! I accused him of being Caesar and Hitler wrapped up in one. (*pause; whimpers again; rocks gently to and fro*) All of a sudden I'm kinda sad. It is sad when your husband has so little understanding of you. Shit! I'm all alone wherever I go. (*crying; pause*)

Crazy, crazy, crazy, crazy! My husband is not tall, he's not beautiful. He doesn't own much hair but you know. . . . In a certain way to some gals he would be attractive and maybe leave me. Why not, I'm such a pain in the rear end. The more I talk, the more I get convinced. Who the hell wouldn't appreciate my life-style. To be married to a successful person. Ah, hell! (*cries; long pause*)

Therapist: I believe the sadness you're experiencing with your husband is a reaction to looking at your mother differently. You were talking about your disappointments with her when you became sad and at that moment reminded yourself of feeling under your husband's thumb. Of a sudden, you felt *he* was the latest tyrant, you to become the oppressed one again. Of a sudden to get along with him, you must submerge yourself again.

Ms. A. R.: I reacting to my mother, to being disappointed at her? No, I'm really disappointed in her. Do I want to be under her thumb? No, I can't stand her small mind, her Betty-Boopishness. She's a throwback to god knows! My brother and I always talk and laugh about her one-liners. She makes Henry Youngman look good. (*pause, begins to whimper*) Why am I sad? It's true, everything I said about her is true. Why am I so sad? (*pause*)

Therapist: When you move away from your mother, this time by facing your differences, you get frightened and want to get under her again. This is what you did with your husband. Suddenly he was the omnipotent one towards whom you submit or rebel. The wish is to dive into the little one under the protection of the queen. It's like you can't be strong with being alone.

Ms. A. R.: Oh, oh, oh, oh! I get it. She hates competition with me. She can't compete, she has to be on stage center. Oh goddammit! I know that, I've always known that, she doesn't want me big! She doesn't want me grown up! (*cries for several minutes*)

I've always whined and complained to her since I was a kid. Maybe until I married. I still do it, as you know. Maybe I do it to get her to attend to business with me. Maybe I learned to do it because of that. It never works. I've told you a thousand times, what does she say? I'm trouble, I *never* get any more from her. (*cries*)

Therapist: You become stronger or get distance from her in any way and then you realize—no mother. You dive back into the little one and you rejoin her, but only if you can be the little one again.

Ms. A. R.: My mother doesn't really love me! Hell, I've always known she has three to four snippy things to say when I show her a new dress or whatever. (*cries*)

I don't know why I call her. Her advice and words are from the Bronze age. I know, you're going to say, I call her to keep me plugged into her, to keep her on the throne.

And so the working through continued with the past-to-the-present movements in psychotherapy, the elaboration of the query, "What is it doing here now?" And the answer that was forthcoming was that "it"—the mother-daughter union—served to keep her in the up-to-now, safe archaic bond with her mother. Growth of her self, and especially growth of her assertiveness, involved separation from her mother, whose mothering had always been totally selective. If she wanted *this* mother she had to posture herself as being without wit or ken. Up to now she had not been able to extricate herself from this defense transference and move on in life. Now, with the awareness of this malignant complex she had the fuel needed to pull herself into the present and recognize that she had to separate herself from living "under" the selfobject as an inadequate self.

After sufficient interpretations of these regressive intrapsychic movements, the patient's capacity to assert herself had become enhanced so she could take those steps that led her away from the mother who could only mirror inferiority. In retrospect her phobia involved a threatened separation from the *archaic* aspect of her mother–daughter dyad, in effect a massive regression. She reexperienced during her phobic phase the maxim that to be without mother was death. Her therapy then was centered on continuing *awareness* of the archaic self/selfobject bond she had entered into then and now. Awareness of this self and its selfobject amounted to mastery of this self of childhood which formerly had, from time to time, dominated the entire psyche.

Phase 4: Termination

Termination in psychoanalytic psychotherapy is the time and situation when the patient and therapist agree that the problem has been sufficiently resolved. The patient's entire self has not been altered, as is hoped for in psychoanalysis. But a considerable amount of relief from the presenting symptoms is to be expected, along with the enhanced functioning of the capacity to observe oneself. Further benefits include the support gained from the self/selfobject relationship of mirroring and calming.

In the case of Ms. A. R. the phobic symptoms had diminished considerably after approximately 24 months—she began to fly again—along with insight into her "attacks" of being the sad, inept little person attaching herself to Queen-like figures. She began discussing after six more months of therapy a wish to be free to go with her husband on further trips and how she missed them. Seeing no resistance she wondered, with the therapist's interest, at the possibility of ending her work sometime in the near future. The therapist stated that, since her problem was now considerably diminished, perhaps in three to four months they could terminate. For about two or three weeks after the discussion on termination she exhibited considerable regressive behavior, the resumption of her symptoms of self-ineptitude.

A segment from the middle of a session during this phase of the therapy (termination) follows:

Ms. A. R.: I was so cool for so long. I haven't had the urge to call my mother and wail. I haven't been beating my husband up for his injustices to poor little me. What's going on? I'm wailing away—someone looks at me funny and I'm all tears. I tried to talk the other day in my literature course and I got all choked up and couldn't continue. What is this? (*cries for several minutes*) Here I am at the end of this therapy and I'm acting like it's the beginning. Boy, is this right? Maybe using medicine would have helped. Do you ever use medicine at this stage? Listen I'm getting worried—this has been going on for a few weeks. You've got to help me. I can't go on like this. You can't just leave me. It's not fair. (*cries with sobs; long pause*)

Therapist: I think we're looking at the old experience of being alone without any comforters during another time of stress.

Ms. A. R.: Words, words, words, words. You're not doing anything. I'm not feeling well, do you understand? (*cries; long pause*) Maybe I was never meant to be together. All that crap I've been through all my life. Don't I deserve some peace? Well, I never get to feel good and strong all the time.

Therapist: Here it is again—the old experience of you in need but unable to stick your arms up and get picked up. This time it's with me. You want *me* to pick you up.

Ms. A. R.: Yes, yes, yes! (*cries*) You're not stopping me *at all*! How will you tell I'm OK? How will you ever know? Am I just another case? You've always stressed empathy and understanding but you're letting me go. How can you be sure? What if I need to come back. What if I fall on my face in the first week after I leave here? (*cries; long pause*) Yes, you're right, you're right. I was feeling that old crap. I'm all alone and feeling blue. Me and my shadow. (*pause*) But still, how can you tell? I may have to call you—I want to call you—you have to keep up with me. (*cries; pause*)

Look how fast this stuff comes up? I'm supposed to be leaving.

Therapist: Your leaving me is experienced as me turning my back on you—as if, as if once again you have legitimate wants and no one—this time me—will respond.

Ms. A. R.: Yes, yes. I got into it again. (*pause*) I feel better. Boy, this is a tough part of the therapy.

As stated above, the return of Ms. A. R.'s experience of being inept was prominent during the first two or three weeks after deciding on a termination date. After this time she continued without incident to the date of termination.

It is very conceivable that this patient will return for the therapy of psychoanalysis since her self was not, in the therapist's view, filled with enough worth or value, the cement of cohesiveness, thus making her vulnerable to future episodes of anxiety or depression.

The next chapter on psychoanalysis will highlight the difference between psychoanalysis and the other forms of therapy. It includes the indications for psychoanalysis, the goals and methods of psychoanalysis, and the hoped-for results.

6

Psychoanalysis

As previously indicated, psychoanalysis is the therapy of choice for those patients who suffer with a self-disturbance—a character disorder—in which so much of their self is disrupted that they cannot engage in either work or play with sufficient emotional gratification. Many of these people with profound self disturbances have an incapacity to form human bonds sufficient to bring them emotional sustenance, although they often are excellent achievers in intellectual or artistic pursuits or in business. Often these patients have attempted one or other forms of psychotherapy which have not been helpful, such as supportive therapy or psychoanalytic psychotherapy. At times, the therapeutic diagnosis of the need for psychoanalysis is made after a course of psychoanalytic psychotherapy is found to be ineffective in producing the desired results towards a self that can form mature self/selfobject bonds and be assertive, love, and be loved.

In sum, the diagnosis of psychoanalysis as the required therapeutic modality is made when a person's self is judged to be unformed in several of its basic structures and functions and that this deficit is chronic, ordinarily a result of a stunted self-development. Further, the indication for psychoanalysis is that the pervasiveness of the self-deficit or character disorder requires a reliving and therefore a reexamining of the patient's earliest self/selfobject relations, i.e., an analysis of the transference, the specific and unique feature of psychoanalysis. As in most character disorders or self disorders, the defective development and therefore defective structuralization is a result of an intense deprivation during a phase of the self's development, usually in childhood, but it may come about in later times of the still-developing self. The diagnosis of the need for analysis may be made only after a period of psychotherapy makes it clear that the specific work of analysis is indicated: the repeated reliving of the archaic self/selfobject encounters in order to eventually cause their impact on the here-and-now interactions to be diminished.

It is this task that psychoanalysis, of all the therapies, performs best since psychoanalysis has as its major mission the furtherance of a so-called therapeutic regression in which the patient begins to experience his therapist as an authority figure and to relive his ungratified needs—those needs and the associated fears and inhibitions that have stifled his ability to grow beyond those periods of deprivation, the fixation points of his self. Once these archaic relationships, the self/selfobject transferences, are formed, the patients begin to reveal to the analyst their previously buried wishes for gratifications appropriate to these childhood periods in which the deprivation occurred. In some patients it will be the need for a selfobject who will calm and soothe; for others it will be for a selfobject who can support (mirror) the assertiveness of a four-year-old through an oedipal phase. Of course, these strivings commonly emerge as defenses *against* these strivings in what we have called a defense transference, in which the patient invests the analyst with the features of his archaic and ungratifying authority figure and then adopts a posture of defense, the protective measures necessary for keeping the intrapsychic peace.

Psychoanalysis has a methodology of data gathering that is unique and integral to the therapeutic transformations. It also has a specific technique for the therapeutic interventions of the analyst. These considerations are part of the clinical theory of psychoanalysis, which is founded on the notion that relived self/selfobject encounters, when illuminated, will enable the patient to now isolate and to ultimately repudiate these archaic appetites and the archaic self/selfobject bonds and go on to develop, with appropriate selfobject support, a self that can be assertive and achieving (Basch, 1981).

In an analysis conducted along self psychology lines, the focus, after the archaic strivings and fixations are diminished, is on the restarted development of the self through the selfobject bond formed with the analyst and the vicissitudes of this bond. As in ordinary development, the self/selfobject bond eventually will result in internalization of the analyst's selfobject functions so that the mirroring functions of the analyst ultimately become internalized as the patient's self experiencing self-worth.

To repeat what has been pointed out earlier, the analysis almost always goes through an initial stage, the formation of a defense transference in which the patient unconsciously views his analyst as a selfobject akin to the selfobjects of his childhood. The patient then experiences those needs, also from childhood, to posture himself in a manner guaranteed to derive optimal gratification or at least safety from this unempathic and potentially dangerous selfobject, the analyst. If the patient and analyst are successful in overcoming this defense transference through interpretations of these patterns and with the ambience of acceptance, the patient will move into the next phase of the transference, the formation of the selfobject transference. The therapeutic bonding of the selfobject transference, whether it be a mirroring, idealized parent or twinship selfobject relationship, will, after internalization of the therapist's selfobject functions, result in the development of his underdeveloped self. Throughout the analysis there will be instances in which the defense transference will reemerge and once again there will be the need to reilluminate this old pattern of defense. In these situations the patient will often, as a result of an empathic failure by the therapist or an uncontrollable narcissistic injury (vacations, illness), revert to the ancient defense against the now-experienced unempathic analyst. The therapist, alerted to these old defense patterns, interprets to the patient that the old archaic pattern is in the room and that, once highlighted and traced to its childhood root, will again be neutralized. However, during the period of *withdrawal* from the analyst—the so-called optimal frustration—there will be a heightened inner experience of the analyst's self and its functions; the *imago* of the analyst through withdrawal from his actual presence will become intensified (Kohut, 1984). This process was first described by Freud to explain the phenomenon of a heightened *inner* experience in the survivor of a person who has been lost through death (Freud, 1917a). These instances of repeated highlighting of these old patterns, which represent on the patient's part the attempt to maintain the old archaic self/selfobject patterns, are called the "working-through" aspects of psychoanalysis (Muslin, 1986).

From the classical psychoanalytic perspective, an analysis is also centered on the uncovering of the childhood relationships and the need to illustrate these resistances to growth through the reliving of these patterns with the analyst—the so-called transference neurosis. In the classical view, however, the transference neurosis will illuminate a central pathological pattern; the oedipal neurosis or a variant of this complex in which the patient's difficulties revolve around the unresolved complex and therefore fixation in his oedipal development. The patient in adult life continues to show difficulties reflecting his continuing fear and inhibitions of his pervasive, albeit unconscious, oedipally centered drives. The defense transference phase of the analysis will ordinarily reflect the patient's *defenses* against these oedipal *drives*, and the analyst ordinarily must strive to make conscious these unconscious defenses so that ultimately the transference will become "oedipal."

A representative defense transference in a classical analysis would reveal the patient showing the preoedipal features of a youngster who is experiencing the analyst in a dyadic manner, i.e., the analyst as a mother figure, the patient as the child. Once the requisite interpretations of this defense pattern are given and effectively utilized, the patient's material, it is held, will begin to show oedipal features in which the patient views the analyst in a variety of manners reflecting the relived oedipal drama, e.g., as a potent destructor who is angry over the patient's assertiveness or sexual prowess (positive oedipal transference). There are many variations of this basic theme but the central issue in classical psychoanalysis is to illuminate through interpretations the pre-oedipal defenses against the pathogenic drives, ordinarily of the oedipal phase of development, in which a significant aspect of the patient's self has become fixated. Subsequent to the neutralization of these defenses, the patient will enter into the transference neurosis which, after sufficient interpretation, will become known to the patient and hopefully evoke memory traces of the original genetic picture. After the patient is able to recognize his childhood complexes both in the transference with the analyst and in the uncovered past, the patient's capacity for here-and-now relationships will then be free from contamination by the ancient oedipal conflicts of the past.

The endpoints of a self psychology analysis are that the patient has resumed his self-development in analysis and now experiences himself with more *worth* through accretion of the mirroring and other self-accretions internalized from the analyst's selfobject functions. Other endpoints are that the patient no longer unconsciously engages in *archaic* self/selfobject encounters but is now enabled to seek out mature human encounters for nurturance and invigoration without hiding behind his defense against the human encounter. In a classical analysis, the endpoints will be that the patient no longer becomes involved in relationships tainted with aspirations and behavior of childhood oedipal sexuality and will be able to be the authentic husband and father. If this complex is not resolved, he will continue in multiple relationships maintained on a superficial level (the Don Juan character). The patient will now be enabled to do what he should have done in childhood: repress his childhood incestuous and destructive strivings towards his mother and father and enter into a life not contaminated with thoughts of incest and retribution from a father-figure.

THE COURSE OF PSYCHOANALYSIS

Phase 1: Rapport, Beginning of Therapeutic Alliance

The analyst introduces the specific data-gathering techniques of analysis: the couch, free association, and the analyst's need to be in a state of abstinence. The patient begins the work of free association with minimal interruptions by the analyst, such as the attempts to encourage the patient to look together (to ally with the analyst) with him at associations that reflect a special pattern important to observe and thereby to evoke more associations, the methodology of psychoanalytic psychotherapy.

Phase 2: Defense Transference, Interpretation

The patient spontaneously begins to experience the analyst as a potentially dangerous or seductive authority figure and concurrently the need to protect himself—he may withdraw, he may become hostile. The analyst is ordinarily called on to interpret this defense posture as an instance of the past-in-the-present with two transference structures emerging: the analyst becomes the significant adult out of the patient's past; the analysand becomes the youngster of his past maintaining distance between himself and the malevolent selfobject.

In self psychology analysis, the interpretation and dissolution of the defense transference ushers in the formation of the therapeutic transference, whichever transference (mirroring, idealized transferring) the patient will spontaneously unfold, a result of his unique fixations. Whenever a significant threat to the therapeutic selfobject bond occurs, the patient reverts back to the defense transference, which offers a bond, albeit a limited and even a painful one.

In classical analysis, as cited above, the defense transference commonly consists of entering into a preoedipal or pregenital experience of the analyst and the analytic relationship in an attempt to fend off the oedipal strivings for incest and parricide. The analyst's interventions will focus on attempts to get the patient to "see" his defenses and help the ushering in of the transference neurosis in which the patient reexperiences his archaic wishes and fears of the oedipal drama.

Phase 3: The Therapeutic Transference

The middle phase of analysis conducted along self psychology lines is ushered in with the formation of a self/selfobject bond, in which the selfobject analyst becomes the purveyor of worth or calming, and ends with the patient experiencing *self-worth*, now enabled to calm himself and be invested with firm interiorized values by which he can be led. In an analysis conducted along classical lines, the middle phase of analysis consists of the transference neurosis, the psychological drama in which the patient enters into a reliving with the analyst of the original traumatic oedipal experience replete with incest wishes and castration fears, parricidal fantasies and dreams. All of the latter represent the archaic contents of the patient's phallic period of development now relived—in fantasy—in the analytic relationship, the analyst being experienced variously as the father-punisher or the mother-seducer. The middle phase of a classical analysis ends after those interpretations that have made his oedipal strivings conscious to the analyst have now evoked the patient's memories of the actual oedipal drama of his childhood. Now the patient can with the analyst *observe* these ancient drives and the associated fears as manifestations of the retained—although until now unconscious—experience of the youngster. These complexes were preserved in their original state through repression as a result of the traumatic circumstances in which the expressions of assertiveness of all kinds on the part of the youngster were not met with empathic-informed acceptance and mirroring, but with hostility. As a result, the ordinary oedipal phase robustness and sexuality became transformed into frightening sexual and aggressive urges that became repressed as they became associated with frightening rejections and even more frightening punitive fantasies, such as fears of castration. The impulses for intimacy and the expressions of assertiveness themselves became taboo and permanently identified with dangerous rejections. As the patient continues to become aware of his identification of his adult drive with the retained experience of the oedipal youngster, these complexes, now remembered in their historical light, can be permanently repressed, no longer attached to the drives for intimacy as evil and taboo instinctual derivatives. This working-through phase comes to an end when as much of the patient's memories of these early phases of his or her life can be unearthed, and the oedipal transference onto the analyst becomes diminished.

The middle phase of the self psychology analysis starts with the spontaneous unfolding of one of the selfobject transferences which pinpoints the specific selfobject dilemma of the patient. As the patient's analysis focuses on the lifelong selfobject needs and distresses in the past and present, the formation of the self/selfobject bond promotes a state of cohesion in the patient which alleviates a great deal of the distresses in the self relating to narcissistic deficits, such as emptiness and loneliness, and enhances the experience of well-being. The specific curative process in self psychology analysis is towards the development of a self that is, when analysis starts, deficient in those structures and functions that maintain the cohesiveness of the self, the endogenous sources of calming and soothing and/or the experiences of self-regard. All these structures and functions emanate from contact with empathic selfobjects in whose presence their functions of mirroring and calming become internalized so as to form endogenous sources of self-worth and self-calming.

In analysis the analyst's selfobject presence in the patient's self-experience promotes the development of those defective self-functions such as the experience of self-worth. The analyst does not "become" the selfobject either by his words or by his actions. It is the patient who transfers onto the analyst the selfobject power and functions derived from the patient's archaic selfobjects, the particular selfobject and its functions with which he is deficient of course and is conflicted over. Now the patient begins to relate to the analyst as the supplicant to the benefactor. The patient experiences the analyst's nonintrusive presence in a beneficent manner as affirming or calming-soothing as he/she freely associates in the analysis from here-and-now events to historical allusions.

However, the positive ambience, the accretion of structure, and the experience of self-calming do not accrue simply from the formation of a self/selfobject bond. For this to occur, the patient's imagoes of the selfobject's functions need to be enhanced or stated differently, sufficiently internalized. As noted previously, this occurs at times through the unavoidable empathic errors or slights or rejection which usher in an optimal frustration followed by a withdrawal. In this withdrawal period the patient's self-memories of the analyst's functions—the imago—will become enhanced.

Another mechanism of internalization of function is through an enhanced positive identification, to "be like" the analyst.

After an adequate period of empathic relatedness, the therapeutic bond ordinarily has developed into a trustworthy institution; now interspersed with the usual amounts of optimal frustration and optimal gratifications, the patient's self *does* go on to develop endogenous stories of well-being, the formation of self-worth and self-calming, and the enhancement of the pole of ideals along with other enhanced self-functions, such as a firmer capacity for maintaining cohesion without fragmentation (Bacal, 1985). Perhaps the most important transformation in the self as a result of psychoanalysis is that of the self's capacity to seek out and not avoid mature selfobjects for nurturance, the process of obtaining psychological oxygen of which Kohut spoke (Kohut, 1971). Another major transformation in the analyzed self is that the patient no longer unconsciously seeks out archaic selfobjects to reenact ancient self/selfobject dramas in which the patient is in effect going through, once again, a defense transference.

Phase 4: The Termination

The essential work done in the crucial termination phase is first to unearth whatever remains of the wishes to enter into archaic self/selfobject encounters and, second, through the process of investigating the remnants of the defense transference, to cause the residue of this complex to become dissolved. The termination phase of an analysis usually involves a telescoping of the entire analysis: rapid and intense movements of regression and forward activity. It is important to have an adequate period of time set aside for the termination period, anywhere from three months to nine months, or even more in complex analyses. The analyst, of course, does not wish to leave the patient in a painful, regressed self-state.

A CASE STUDY

The following case study will demonstrate a case of a self psychology analysis. We will consider the analysis of the case of Ms. B. C. first described for purposes of diagnosis earlier in this volume (pp. 55–59). We will begin by summarizing the pertinent history, including the indications for psychoanalysis.

Pertinent History (Summarized)

Ms. B. C. came to this analysis after experiencing a depression which had many antecedents. Her most recent stressor was in the mourning for her father, then dead one year. Her second child had been born four months prior to her entering this analysis. In the background she was still in mourning for her mother who had died 12 years previously.

She described her childhood, adolescence, and early adulthood as filled with deprivations and sadness. Several events stood out in her infancy and childhood that militated against an ordinary development. She had been told many times that she was colicky and could not be calmed. In her view she never experienced her mother as a source of warmth or nurturance; she found herself fearful (already in her third year) of being picked up by her mother, which she always associated with the rejection of quickly putting her in her crib or putting her down without further contact. As she became older, the pattern continued of walling herself off from mother, fearing either coldness or criticism. She entered elementary school as an agitated and lonely person already a victim of the unconscious equation of closeness equaling abandonment.

Her father, towards whom she always felt more positively, did try to engage her in his leisure activities but it was too late in her development to compensate for the primary maternal (mirroring) deprivation. Her father remained in her experience as an idealized person from afar who did not utilize his capacities to guide her in any of her activities.

Her experiences of high school continued to be dominated by her need to remain isolated from her fellow students and her professors. She did not enter into any social activities nor did she have dates with men. From the time she was 15 she became chronically depressed; four years later it was discovered that her mother had a cancer of the breast. The patient began her psychotherapy (age 15) and later psychoanalysis (age 20) in reaction to her own increasingly painful sadness and agitation.

Her first analysis started directly after her mother's death and was, as she stated, "all about my Oedipus complex, the wish to dethrone my mother and possess my father." She did also receive help in diminishing her fear of men and began going to parties and dances. She met her husband at a dance and shortly afterwards married him. Their marriage was marred by her lifelong difficulty in being receptive to intimacy.

Her presenting self-state was that of an agitated, lonely 32-year-old woman experiencing the painful self-state that is associated with a loss of self-worth. The empathic diagnosis was that she was suffering from a narcissistic deficit disorder with an enfeebled self, seemingly without any endogenous supplies of esteem. She seemed to be without a capacity to calm herself. The therapeutic diagnosis was that since she was experiencing difficulties in so many facets of her life, she would require psychoanalysis. It was, of course, noted that she was able to enter into a therapeutic relationship in the past and had derived benefit from her analysis.

Review of the Analysis

In a nutshell, as Kohut often said, the entire analysis concerned itself with the vicissitudes of the patient's fixation on a life of restraint and vigilance towards potential invaders of her life space. Her previous work in analysis had not given her either the knowledge or experiences necessary to extricate her from her self of isolation, a self filled with fears of being touched and therefore filled with barricades to intimacy in many forms—towards mirroring, towards calming, towards being led. Her fixations onto this self had led to her experience of life as being empty, but she was unaware that she was functionally unable to enjoy the supports which were offered from her milieu—she was filled with "empty complaints," i.e., complaints that she could not pursue further to gratification. Many other methods of maintaining this self of isolation became evident through the analysis—dueling with the analyst, withholding information, curtailing the length of her sessions by coming late and leaving early.

The analysis began with the patient expressing fear of allowing the analyst to enter into her psychic life in a manner exactly similar to her first analysis, at least in her view. Further, she stated that her behaviors and even her voice seemed the same. From the analyst's point of view, he witnessed a person remarkably responsive to any movement on his part, to which she would react with intense anxiety. During the first years of analysis, her voice would approach the intensity of shrieking. Her anxiety, centered on her responses to the analyst, dictated that the analysis focus on her immediate entry into the defense transference in which the analyst was experienced as the agent of punishment. The analyst quickly learned that his task was to provide a milieu without overt interventions so that she would begin to experience a safe environment over a long period of time, free from any unprecipitated "controlling" on the analyst's part.

Little by little the manner in which she structured her life emerged; as alluded to previously, she managed to keep everyone, emotionally speaking, at bay. Although she appeared to have many complaints about her unfulfilled longings, complaints, as mentioned above, could not proceed to fulfillment since the posture of receptivity required could not be experienced without panic. She attended to all of her "duties" pro forma without joy since the pathway to discharge of her strivings was stunted. In this way she maintained herself—empty, lonely, but safe. She began now, of course, to repeat this defensive pattern to the analyst with complaints of loneliness and defenses against gratification sometimes with nonverbal behaviors (latecoming, early leaving) and other times with verbal behaviors (such as rejections of any and all of the analyst's comments). The analyst was sometimes able, at first very tentatively and infrequently, to explain the repetitiousness in her experience of the analyst as another potential imprisoner.

At the end of the second year, she responded to these interventions and the analytic milieu by recounting the history (the actual memories) of her early days with her mother—the fear of her embraces—and those early fears of being cast away were reconstructed. Over the next long period of time, this archaic pattern of protection waned and the patient began to experience, not just complaints of the analyst's indifference, but direct wishes for more and more comforts from analysis.

Finally, the actual experiences of being calmed emerged in the analysis. The patient now revealed that her mothering patterns had changed—she could now touch and hold her children and husband. There were a variety of changes in her life that were also manifest—from asking for warmth from her husband to resuming contacts with her siblings that had previously been avoided. In analysis, she could now enter into the work with enthusiasm since, as she said, she was no longer anticipating "putdowns" which had blocked her in the past. Now the work centered more and more on the emergence of assertive strivings, which was quickly followed by the psychological "looking backwards" to see if the analyst was still there and approving. Then there was usually a dip into the old experience of empty complaining, followed by a return to the here-and-now benevolent milieu of analysis. A typical pattern would be that of telling the analyst about a weekend with her husband in which she had a love experience with him that was "good," followed by associations to worries of an impending separation from the analyst and then to an experience of a sad memory of bringing her mother a homework assignment only to have it taken over by her mother. Finally, she would "wake up" and remind herself of the distance between then and now.

When the patient announced that she now wished to terminate, it seemed to be a reasonable decision. She had over the past two years been able to engage in her life pursuits with enthusiasm, free from her previous shackles of restraint. As mother, wife, and friend, she now seemed to consistently excel. In her analysis, there was little evidence of either the old defense patterns or the exquisite sensitivities to interruptions or empathic errors by retreat into defense patterns.

The Termination Phase

The sessions directly after the setting of the termination date found Ms. B. C. in a state of painful agitation. She was frightened over separating from analysis, coupled with her experiences that the analyst was not sufficiently involved with her and that she was being dismissed because of disappointment with her performance in analysis. These comments evoked associations to her mother, whose interest in her emerged only when she was in great need, indeed when she clamored or actually fought for attention. No fighting or clamoring, no attention. On the other hand, since childhood she had been uneasy around her mother, fearing physical contact with her. The interpretations that the analyst made at this point, one month after the date setting for termination, were that she was structuring her relationship in analysis so that the analyst would stop the termination or *make* her come to her treatment indefinitely. Her subsequent associations to this interpretation confirmed the latter.

Thus, directly after the date of termination was set, the patient's experience of the analyst heightened considerably and led to a restructuring of her relationship in analysis so that the analyst was witness to the defense transference that was prominent in the earlier part of her analysis. In this defense transference, the patient's experience of the analyst was that he was withdrawn, withholding, and unempathic. This pattern of Ms. B. C. defending herself was previously reconstructed in her analysis as having two roots. One was traced to her mother who had many periods in which she was aloof and distracted and unavailable to her children. Second, at times she experienced her mother as a frightening presence who might imprison her. In her early life, she had been a colicky infant and could not be calmed. She had never experienced her mother's embraces as soothing, only as leading to isolation in her crib, without relief of pain. Thus her need to experience the analyst suddenly as a non-giver expressed the defense against painful isolation, a residue of her infancy, as well as expressive of the defense from childhood against being hurt by exposing wants and needs that would not be gratified.

Now suddenly, so it seemed, after the initial post-date-setting phase of the heightened defense transference, a break in this mode of interaction transpired and the patient became again receptive to the presence and the words of the analyst and experienced calming and enhanced worth without resistance. For the remainder of the months of Ms. B. C.'s termination process, this pattern—the resumption of her defense transference and the working through of this pattern, followed by the acceptance of the analyst's interest and the enhancing of her self-value and cohesiveness—repeated itself.

In the next month of her analysis, Ms. B. C.'s defense transference was again reenacted in relation to her husband and their three children. Once again she "had" to be the cement of the family, obeying only what she interpreted as their needs and her role in gratifying these needs: "He's not like my partner; I have to take care of everything. It's me taking care of myself again. No one is on my side. I never felt anyone on my side—my younger sister, my younger brothers. Now my children and my husband." And then on the following day of the analysis, she would say: "I had to tell you how terrible it was, regardless of what you were saying or doing. I still want you to hear how bad it's been." On this same following day, she would experience and articulate the idea that she had been very much helped by the analyst's presence in sharing and understanding her burdens from the past and present.

The analyst did, during this time, have occasion to interpret to her that he, too, was experienced as a non-giver and that she was, in effect, dismissing him and not deriving any support from him. These comments liberated memories of her years of caretaking of a cancer-ridden mother and a well-meaning but ineffectual father, and a vivid—previously repressed—memory of the death scene of her mother. The analyst's comments pertaining to her transference onto him as yet another non-giver evoked the patient's experience that he, too, overvalued her capacities as a caretaker and in this way he, too, was not genuinely appreciating her.

At the end of this intense period of reliving the experience of being unappreciated, unrecognized, only living for others—her "rightful place in the sun"—Ms. B. C. quietly expressed the feeling that she would miss her analysis, the help she derived from sharing her inner life. In fact, she became uneasy, stating, "How do I do without you? What am I going to do when I quit seeing you?" These statements revealed that, temporarily at least, the patient was once again experiencing the analyst as the actual provider of self-worth, that no internalizations had taken place, and that no structural defect had been overcome.

The next sessions were filled with Ms. B. C.'s ongoing complaints that she was going to have a difficult time without her analysis, but indeed her associations revealed that she was continuing in the revival of the defense transference and again isolating herself. There followed sessions in which she felt somewhat calmed and soothed but continued to complain that she would be " . . . frightened. I'll stop growing if I don't see you for you to tell me all these things. Only recently I've been able to hear you. I can't remember enough from you." She complained of not being able to tell the analyst of her wants. The process revealed her struggle in these intensified and *telescoped* episodes of experiencing herself as *only* being able to complain that she was not appreciated and being needy of guidance, support, and cherishing, *but* actually being unable to extricate herself from the repetitive clutches of her defense transference so as to *experience* the calming of her basic self/selfobject transference in which she had formerly been.

The struggle continued with the alternating sessions of experiencing herself in despair, *only* able to complain over a non-giving husband and a difficult home situation, in contrast to sessions where she, of a sudden regaining her basic transference and her cohesive self, felt in equilibrium but still complained that it would not be sufficient to maintain her equilibrium in the future. These alternative self-states began to follow a pattern of one session in which she was at peace, followed by the next session in which she would, for example, dream of an ancient scene of feeling abandoned in a private high school. Her associations led to the feeling that the analyst was betraying her by allowing her to terminate. The interpretations of this defensive pattern, with the analyst alternately as the ungiving and potentially frightening selfobject mother and the indifferent father allowing her to wallow in a sea of unresponsiveness, did allow her to review again the data of her childhood deprivations and fears.

The next period—the final month—dealt with Ms. B. C.'s feeling flooded by her wishes to permanently attach herself to the analyst. She felt that coming to analysis was crucial and she was distressed at the prospect of losing the analyst and not having a replacement for him. This expression of the analyst's importance to her, and the stated experience of the analysis being for her and centered on the appreciation of her, was a new element for her which had developed in the analysis. The grief that seemed to be in view at this time was focused on her separation from analysis— without displacements now—and highlighted in a dream of aloneness:

> I had an appointment to see you in a large foreign city. There was a sudden burst of rain on the city, stopping traffic. I could hardly see through the window from my car. I stopped to ask a policeman for directions; it was two miles in the opposite direction. I decided to walk, and suddenly in front of me I saw an awesome church which made me stop and view it in wonder. The Vatican? St. Paul's? I woke up before I could see you.

The awesome church made her think of the overpowering feeling of loss of the analysis and the analyst without replacements. The other associations dealt with the grief of "feeling you inside of me and now it's going to hurt to lose you."

The last three weeks were a mixture of complaints of not feeling well, feeling incomplete, and questioning why she had to leave. The analyst repeated the familiar interpretations to her of her wish to leave analysis as a sad, deprived person still living out her life with the experiences of being unvalued. She had had a series of dreams all relating to the theme of being with a person (man) who rejected her, which were the data that initiated the analyst's repetitive interpretation. She complained at length over her inability to celebrate her achievement in terminating the analysis and related it to her mother who was never present for her triumphs in school or elsewhere. Ms. B. C. said, "I've changed unbelievably; it's hard to remember what I was like. I'm so different in my self-esteem. I just don't have problems anymore. I've just not felt cherished in *here.*" The tension of experiencing the intense relived deprivation during one session evoked in her a cry for help that the analyst was not providing. She had had a dream in which a friend needed financial aid. She went to the bank and talked the loan officer into

giving her friend a loan. Her associations to this dream culminat-
ed in her awareness that she needed the analyst to be her advo-
cate. She said, "Why am I having this dream now? I'm not starting, I'm terminating."

Finally, three sessions before the end, Ms. B. C. recounted that
the "sad period is over." All the relived pain of deprivation was
seemingly at an end and a mixture of pleasurable feelings and
sadness now finished the analysis. She had a triumphal dream in
which she was singled out by a man and in the process "outshone
the other woman who was competing for him." However, as she
stated, "The other woman without anger recognized it." She said
in her elaboration and interpretation of the dream, "They both felt
good about me. I didn't have any ulterior motive. I just didn't
have to hold back. I felt recognized for my worth." She associated
to the lifelong pattern of her unrewarded and guilt-ridden strivings for outclassing her mother, which were finally resolved in the
dream. The next material dealt with her sadness that life would be
difficult without the analyst to know about her and to recognize
her accomplishments. And then came the last session.

The last session began with a gift, a wall hanging that Ms. B. C.
said would remind the analyst of her. She then recounted her final
dream:

> I was standing in a line at a local store. Actually I felt I was
> observing myself. Suddenly there was my mother's fur jack-
> et in front of me and I tried it on in front of a mirror. It looked
> good on me.

Ms. B. C. said, "It was the first time I ever put together my mother
and myself. I just realized I had my hair up like she wore it at
times." She associated to wanting to hear "parting words of wisdom" from the analyst and when he told her that just as in the
dream she looked good to him, she commented that her husband
was also pleased at her progress. She felt calmed but then wondered how the analyst was experiencing her leave taking. She
associated then to a time when her mother wanted to live with her
permanently after a visit in college which caused her distress. She
discounted the analyst's comment that she was harboring a con-

cern over whether he was genuinely pleased over her sprouting wings by telling him that she knew he was pleased "without strings attached." She said, "I've never been able to feel important and special. I've gotten enough. I have tools to straighten myself out if I get down. I guess I've grown up. We haven't left anything out."

DISCUSSION

The discussion will center on three major issues: the indications for analysis; the goals for self-transformations in analysis; and the contrast between the goals in an analysis and the other psychotherapies. However, an overview of the work performed in the analysis of Ms. B. C. and the subsequent self-transformations are considered first.

In the description of the analysis it was clear that the patient became caught up in the selfobject transference in which she sought self-nurturance to correct her lifelong experience of an enfeebled self. As Freud (1917b) emphasized many years ago, the transference is the "battleground" of the analysis. As will be recalled, Ms. B. C. entered into her therapeutic transference (the idealized selfobject transference) through a lengthy passageway of the defense transference. Her main experience of the analyst for many months (over two years) was that the analyst—like her mother—was not appreciative of her, not empathic of her self-needs, and that he was a potential imprisoner and abandoner, not a safe person to unfold one's heartfelt needs to. Her "defense" to this transference was to relate—mimicking her original reaction to her mother and her childhood environment—as a youngster struggling for her life against those who would imprison her.

The illumination of this defense transference was a crucial part of the analysis as it helped extricate her from years of bondage to an archaic and painful posture, the self of the inept and alone youngster to which she repetitiously turned as if *all* human encounters were potentially imprisoning. The compulsion to repeat, to restructure, the tragic maternal self/selfobject dyad *on her part*, especially the entry into the self of subservience, had to be illuminated several times over many months until there was adequate self-splitting to enable the patient to "see" the archaic self occupy center stage. This self posture of being combative and secretive and not able to directly unfold her needs represented an invaluable method of security maintenance in living with her mother. However, this type of defense pattern was inimical to any here-and-now mature self interests.

The repeated interpretations of the defense transference, the double transference onto the analyst and the patient, resulted in the awareness on the patient's part of this repetitious pattern of interacting that kept her imprisoned. Her associations to her past helped her to gain an awareness of the stifling addictive aspects of this pattern. Directly after, her material revealed that she was less involved in the setting up of those scenes where she would be deprived and demeaned as she began to experience a self/selfobject dyad that eventually led to her accreting the necessary self-structures for an adaptive life: an enhanced experience of self-worth, an enhanced capacity to assert herself, especially in the form of seeking out others to be of service to herself.

As will be remembered, these positive self-changes were observed, by contrast, in a highly dramatic fashion during Ms. B. C.'s termination when the archaic self-patterns were once again in the forefront and her defense transference again occupied center stage. Once again the analyst *became* the not-to-be-trusted deliverer of punishment.

Now let us consider the issue of the indications for psychoanalysis in contrast to the other therapies. A related question is to the hoped-for self-changes in analysis—what should be the goals in psychoanalysis *and* are they accomplished *only* in analysis?

We have already indicated that psychoanalysis is the psychotherapy of choice when the self is so riddled with deficits that ordinary activities cannot be performed without a variety of painful experiences related to an enfeebled self: doubting, demeaning, and ineptitude. We have also stated that those in need of and who will benefit from analysis clearly cannot be in a state of crisis-fragmentation. Psychoanalysis is the therapy reserved for those whose *selves* are not in distress in reaction to a particular environment; rather it is their abiding perceptions and reactions that cause their distress. The former situation represents the need

for supportive psychotherapy and the latter situation for psychoanalytic psychotherapy. Those patients who require analysis or are
best served by analysis have selves that do not "work": these are
selves that cannot provide requisite gratifications to ensure equilibrium regardless of the environment in which they find themselves. There is not enough assertiveness to seek out human
sources of calming or admiration or there is so much resistance to
the human input of warmth that the end result of loneliness continues. So often in those who require psychoanalysis their endogenous stores of ideals which fuel action are missing, leaving those
without these internalized ideals to continually seek out leaders to
follow who ultimately disappoint, as they cannot satiate the intense needs of these ideal-empty selves. Moreover, the overall
selves of those who require analysis, with their self-functions and
selfobject strivings, are found to be fixed in the form of their selves
of childhood when the self-development became impeded. Thus
they seek to engage others in a continual repetition of their original self/selfobject bonds, looking for the mirroring or the calming
that was left out of their early life. As noted above, these are
patients whose self-functions of observing and repression are
wanting.

As a necessary consequence of these profound and pervasive
self disturbances which so interfere with current functioning, the
psychotherapist should consider a referral of these patients to the
analyst. It is in analysis that the pervasive self-disorder will be
enabled to become transformed. This is the goal of analysis:

> Psychoanalysis has as its goal that the self will be trans-
> formed: significantly more assertiveness will be manifest;
> there will be selfobjects sought after for human succor in
> time of need; and there will be more in the way of ideals
> experienced, through which the self will be led to greater
> achievements. The entire activities of the self will be devoted
> in part to the pursuit of a joyous existence.

The essentials of the cure in analysis are based in no small way
on the reliving and reexamining of the early pathogenic scenes
now transferred onto the analyst and the analyst/analysand rela-

tionship. Ultimately, these toxic transferences will be revealed and deenergized so that the patient can accept the analyst and his/her ministrations of acceptance and admiring in order to internalize the analyst's selfobject functions and experience self-worth and self-admiring, the endpoint of an analysis designed to promote the growth of the self. And so in those patients with the chronic, pervasive, tragically enfeebled selves we have described, the repeated immersion into the reliving of their archaic needs and the defenses against these needs within the transference *are* ultimately the preferred and perhaps the only route to the denouement of their self-weaknesses.

There are a number of important requirements of the patient who is in need of analysis. The candidate for analysis cannot be in a state of fragmentation and obtain any benefit from the analysis, based as it is on the patient freely associating the contents of his or her inner life to the therapist who is in a state of abstinence. For an analysis to proceed, the patient must have an optimal capacity for introspection and empathy and with it a well-developed capacity for trust, indicating that the *entire* self cannot be in an unformed state for the work of analysis. Although the diagnosis of the capacity to self-observe and form a therapeutic alliance can be made, the prediction of whether or not the patient will have a "workable transference" is a difficult and often impossible task. An "unworkable transference" is one in which the patient has what Freud would call an "adhesiveness" of the libido (Freud, 1937), indicating a patient's libidinal fixation to one or other of the pregenital phases and therefore the inability to develop beyond these developmental periods. Our focus in a self psychology analysis is on the self/selfobject fixations; our query is whether or not these self/selfobject fixations are too "adhesive" and therefore the self is incapable of further development to part from their archaic bonds. It turns out that there are instances in psychoanalysis when a particular patient's selfobject fixations are, as Freud lamented, interminable, i.e., not capable of change (Freud, 1937).

The final issue in this chapter is the specificity of goals in psychoanalysis. As indicated, the aspirations for analysis are to transform a self that is in distress into a cohesive self through the following: 1) isolating the defense transference and helping diminish it as a defense against a therapeutic bond, and 2) the therapeutic transference with its ultimate outcome of *internalization* of the analyst's mirroring or other selfobject function. Although much internalization occurs in *any* psychotherapy, this is *not* the *goal* for a problem-oriented approach or a supportive approach. Psychoanalysis is the approach to the self-problem that is impacting on many or all aspects of the patient's life. In those cases where sector or psychoanalytic therapy seems the therapy of choice, the therapist has concluded that his patient's overall self-cohesiveness apart from the problem area is not threatened and that he can proceed to isolate the sector for study and clarification as we have indicated. The patient requires the therapist as an ally throughout psychoanalytic psychotherapy, thus precluding any detailed scrutiny of his experiences towards the analyst.

We will now turn to a discussion of the inner life of the therapist and its influence on the work of psychotherapy.

7

The Inner World of the Psychotherapist

The inner world of the psychotherapist is comprised of: 1) *the work self*, those self-experiences and functions related to the mission of establishing and maintaining psychic peace in others, as well as pointing their way to higher states of well-being; and 2) *the subjective self*, being all the remaining thoughts and feelings which attest to the personhood of the therapist. Included in these latter reactions are those of the therapist's *transferences* onto the patient and the countertransferences.

The therapist, as a reactive human entity, experiences his self-reactions to his environment, including his patients, with greater or lesser intensity, reflecting his self at a given time and the quality and quantity of human stimuli. However, the therapist must erect and maintain a barrier against these modal experiences in order to perform his functions as the scientific observer—cognitive and empathic—of the patient. At times the therapist is caught up with self-experiences relating to a variety of preoccupations which strains his capacity to erect this wall and function as an empathic observer. The ideal therapist who remains in empathic harmony with the patient's self-state, while carefully following the details of an interview throughout the entire encounter, remains as our standard, although we realize how often it is an unattainable goal. Consider the situation in which a therapist-in-training who has to listen and gather the data and interact with the patient in sympathy with the precepts of his/her current supervisor, in addition to all of the other ordinary interferences with listening and responding. Consider the inner world of a therapist who is enervated for any number of reasons ranging from chronic illness to an episode of diminished self-esteem but who, nonetheless, must continue performing for extended periods. Consider the inner world of a therapist who is apprehensive over a relative's or colleague's illness. All these situations make the capacity to maintain the "therapist's therapeutic split" difficult and, at times, seemingly impossible. Moreover, these reactions in the therapist's inner world are common for all therapists and not a manifestation of dysfunction in a particular therapist. The dysfunction would surface in those instances in which the therapist's ability to maintain the split is strained to the point that the inner preoccupations of the therapist invade the work self of the therapist and the patient is now witness to spontaneous, unfiltered responses from the therapist.

Once the therapeutic split of the therapist is effected, the therapist's capacity for introspection of the subjective experiences evoked in therapy can be observed and utilized as data; for example, towards the understanding of the patient's impact on his/her environment. Further, the therapist's capacity to draw out formerly buried self-states in himself for empathic purposes is then enhanced, the process which Kohut referred to as the empathy of an individual for himself (Kohut, 1984).

THE WORK SELF

The work self of the therapist comprises all the experiences of the therapist as he observes, assembles, and responds in tune with the required therapeutic activity determined by the patient's need. At times this self must become altered in its psychological shape to perform certain therapeutic functions. This is the case, for example, when the therapist becomes the supportive therapist with a physically ill or terminally ill patient. In this situation there is a need to perform mirroring and other selfobject functions which are aimed at helping the patient in his or her need to maintain a flagging sense of worth. The shape of the self of the therapist in this instance becomes altered so as to become the needed selfobject for this patient's self-needs. In other therapeutic situations, the self-modifications require that the self become an empathizing instrument over long periods of time as is the case in all intensive psychotherapies.

In each of these activities of the work self—from observing to responding—the self is required to exhibit certain functions in response to the diagnosed therapeutic needs. However, selves vary in their capacities to mirror or direct reflecting the individual developmental accents of the individual therapists. These are *not* countertransference reactions; they are developmental differences resulting in structural differences. Psychotherapists vary widely in their capacity to mirror, to act as guides, and to share in feelings. Psychotherapists vary widely in their need to be recognized, i.e., to become included in the patient's inner world; the intensity of this need defines and delimits the capacity to remain as empathic observers when such is required.

THE SUBJECTIVE SELF

The subjective self of the psychotherapist designates the non-therapeutic self and its experiences and activities. The nontherapeutic experiences of a therapist comprise the "civilian" reactions of the therapist to his environment, including the patient with whom he is interacting. These experiences and activities simply refer to the inner world of perceptions and sensations *not* under the sway of the work self, i.e., *not* organized into a self operating in accordance with its ideal of being the empathically tuned instrument in the service of maintaining the patient's cohesion. The transference of the therapist to his patient is one such "civilian" reaction. It comprehends the idea that the psychotherapist in his transference reaction now experiences his patient as a transference object or selfobject. In reaction to his now-transformed self, the therapist looks forward to, becomes apprehensive about, or has a variety of experiences attesting to his anticipation of the patient as a selfobject or object. The therapist's freedom in performing as an empathic instrument will necessarily be restricted as his transferences intrude, outside of his awareness, into his empathic functioning. The transference of the therapist of course becomes altered as a function of the therapist's insight into this transference. Once insight is attained, the therapist has yet another opportunity to work through those residues of his transference, this time not targeted onto *his own* therapist but onto the patient.

Another aspect of the inner world of the therapist is the reactions that are experienced *after* the patient begins his investment onto the therapist of his particular aspirations and anxieties of the past, the so-called therapeutic transferences. Therapists vary widely in their capacity to be the recipient of different transferences or defense transferences and vary in their capacity to maintain "the therapist's therapeutic split." These are the countertransference reactions and, in the narrow sense in which we are using the term, indicate that the therapist is experiencing a reaction to the patient's transference onto him. In this sense it describes an intrapsychic event which is in process ubiquitous, in content idiosyncratic. The outcome of these sequences in the ideal should be an awareness on the therapist's part that a special reaction has taken place to some aspect of the patient or to the patient's material. Our clinical literature is filled with instances of countertransference reactions undetected until the therapist revealed them through actions of one sort or another that were commonly untoward or unhelpful to the progress of the treatment (Racker, 1957). There are other instances reported in the literature in which the countertransference reactions ultimately led to clarification of the patient's transference reactions (Kohut, 1971; Racker, 1957; Tower, 1956).

At bottom, so to speak, the countertransference reactions represent the unfolding of the therapist's uniqueness and thus again reveal the therapist's unique self bringing to *this* therapy his sensitivities and vulnerabilities, as well as his dedication and talents. Although it is obvious that the patient's communications are evo-

cative of some reaction to anyone in his surroundings, the therapist's responses are of course a result of the evocative stimulus
and the therapist's reactive self. Thus, whether early or late in the
therapy (Gitelson, 1952), whatever the material is or is not, the
therapist's self or intrapsychic responses are (one might say, of
course) the crucial experiences in determining the reactions of the
therapist.

The preceding points can now be summarized as follows: Regardless of how much or little obtains in the way of stimulus from
his patient, the therapist experiences special reactions reflecting
his situation at that moment. His final responses and expressions
of his responses will be multidetermined, the end result of the
stimuli from the patient in concert with his self-functioning at that
moment, especially his self-observing functions. These self-reactions are to be understood as those that all therapists in some way
experience. These reactions "clutter up" the therapist's self-observing and self-responding so as to interfere or at least make
difficult the task of focusing on the patient. And, of course, if the
therapist's transference reactions continue to be mainly unconscious, they can and do exert a major impact on the therapist's
behaviors. Immediately, the patient is no longer viewed as a patient caught up in his or her transference neurosis; rather, the
patient has become part of the therapist's transference structuring, a malevolent competitor on a mission of revenge exactly
similar to, say, the dominant sibling of one's past, or the patient is
suddenly experienced not as a patient in a transference, but as an
older female authority figure out of one's past who is demeaning
the defenseless therapist.

In some psychotherapy situations, the therapist's inner world
may similarly become filled with nontransferential love or hate
strivings towards the patient akin to the transferences described
above; these may become pervasive throughout the therapy or
may amount to one or two episodes of expression. These reactions
attest to the discovery that the patient has suddenly become for
this therapist an "ordinary" person, who will be reacted to only
on the basis of his or her perceived manifest behavior as an attractive or outrageous person, offering the possibility of a love-en-

counter or evoking hostility. In this setting, one patient is experienced as uplifting, another as disagreeable, the third as "so attractive," and so on. These reactions may or may not be "caught" by the therapist and therefore not recognized as a retreat from the therapeutic mission. In each case, these reactions *do* represent unfiltered wishes to engage the patient in a negative or positive manner as one does a prospective girlfriend or boyfriend. And, as in an encounter with a girlfriend, there are hidden transference longings for the woman to be not just a source of peer gratification but a source of archaic mirroring as well. These reactions therefore represent strivings that are not contained by the demands of the work self. These strivings are rarely acted on; for the most part a therapist's subjective strivings towards his patient are present in the self as a fantasy and represent yet another set of experiences which further "clutter up" the work self. Rarely does it happen that a therapist will be unable to ultimately contain his negative or positive "nontherapeutic" experiences towards a patient.

How are these unusual happenings in therapy to be explained? To begin with, it is clear that such unbridled and unfettered reactions in a therapist as described represent a special intrapsychic alteration. The therapist's devotion to his mission is ordinarily sufficient to keep him safe from any "civilian"-type responses of a negative or positive nature towards his patient. To be sure, no therapist is ever totally free from these human responses to a person who is suddenly desired as a companion or to whom one experiences revulsion. In most instances, the therapist sooner or later "wakes up" to these intrusive experiences and then continues to work without being distracted by these now neutralized self-strivings to be recognized, to be adulated, and/or to discharge affection or rage. However, in some therapies, the therapist's mission is overridden for variable periods by his object and/or selfobject needs, i.e., his need to be nurtured or cherished, or his previously contained rage at being drained or manipulated in this or other relationships, or his longings for intimacy. The self-transformation is that the work self of the therapist is replaced by the therapist's self-in-need to the patient as the experienced selfobject, mature or archaic, or to the patient as object with a particular self who is desired for his/her special qualities.

As noted, these intrusions into the therapist's self—the transferences as well as the nontransference reactions—may never become conscious, may be carried out in action (acting-out), or may be "caught," introspected, and become part of the "analytic toilet" (Glover, 1928). Perhaps the most cogent overview of the etiology of these intrusions and collapses of the work self is that the work self cannot maintain its integrity when there are major repeated distractions in a therapist's life. Among these distractions are the physiological variables of acute and chronic illness and fatigue which interfere with the capacity of the work self to be cohesive and to continue the mission of being immersed in the patient's self. Other distractions to the work self are those self-deficits of an acute or chronic nature that render the therapist highly vulnerable and reactive to his own self-needs for cherishing or calming. These same self-deficits may render the therapist more reactive to rebuffs, including the rebuffs of a haughty, demeaning patient in a defense transference, or the insults of a paranoid person, or the chronic rebuffs of a complaining, chronically depressed patient.

Some examples from the writings of psychotherapy authors will illustrate the ubiquity and the complexity of the intrusions into the work self of the therapist.

Example 1 (from Freud)

> Persuasive evidence of a transference is contained in the meeting between Freud and Dora when Dora came to see Freud fifteen months after the treatment was over. He says that she came to ask for help, but "one glance at her face, however, was enough to tell me that she was not in earnest over her request." How he possibly could have told this from one glance at her face remains a mystery, and, indeed, the evidence he subsequently gives to indicate that she was not in earnest is unconvincing.
>
> She said that she had come for help with her right-sided facial neuralgia, and when he asked how long it had been

going on, she said, "two weeks." Freud said that he couldn't help smiling, and he was able to show her that two weeks before she had read some news about him in the newspaper. Strachey tells us that this was no doubt news of Freud's appointment to a professorship.

But how do we know what this news meant to her? Even though Freud says he did not know what she wanted, he offers the explanation that her facial neuralgia was a self-punishment, remorse for having given Herr K. a box on the ear and at having transferred her feelings of revenge to him. Despite the fact that Dora had come on her own, rather than, as at first, at her father's bidding, Freud says nothing about the possibility of her positive attachment to him nor does he recognize any genuine desire for help. It may be that his own positive transference led him to reject the implicit wish in her seeking him out—i.e., to renew their relationship. In any event, Freud apparently terminated the interview quickly and never saw her again. (Muslin & Gill, 1978)

Example 2 (from Gitelson)

At the beginning of an hour in a going analysis, a young male patient commented to me that I looked tired. I myself was not aware of fatigue. Towards the end of the hour which he had spent talking about his University activities, he requested a change in the time of his appointment two weeks hence, when he was scheduled to present a paper in a seminar. I responded that I would see what I could do about changing the time. He then retracted his request, giving as his reason that it would inconvenience me. I told him, however, that the request seemed valid and that I would see what change I could make in his appointment. He left my office looking preoccupied.

The next day he brought the following dream:

He has an engagement with his mother but it seems to be incidental to a date which he has later with his mistress.

> He acts as if he were indifferent to his mother and is
> hurried in disposing of the business with her.

The patient then spoke of how upset he felt after the previous hour. I told him that I had noticed it. Then he spoke
about not writing home and about his childhood feeling that
he was incidental to his mother's career interests. His further
comments made it clear that he now ignored the existence of
his parents as he had himself felt ignored. Then he referred
to my "insistence" on rearranging my programme for him,
even after he felt that he had detected some hesitancy on my part.

At this point something recurred to me which I had until
then forgotten: On the morning of the day of my patient's
request, I had arrived earlier than usual at the hospital for the
purpose of discussing cases with the residents. None of them
was around and none appeared until I was about to leave
with only a limited time in which to reach my office. They
had been disappointed because I could not stay on to work
with them. I myself had been irked by their lateness and had
commented on it. But the matter had apparently slipped
from my mind.

I shall not go into the personal ramifications of this episode. But it was clear to me that I had displaced my reaction
in the hospital situation to my office and that my patient had
detected my latent annoyance with him. I did the only thing I
felt I could do: I brought the episode into the open and
admitted the irritation which I recognized I had produced,
without awareness, against him. It developed, however, that
what had affected him most was that he had correctly observed my compensatory attitude. This had impressed him
as a concern for something in myself rather than for him.
That this was more important than my apparent annoyance
with him was shown when he told me that his mother had
often said that she was doing something for his good when
the fact was that it was something in which she had a personal stake. (Gitelson, 1952, pp. 6–7)

Example 3 (from Tower)

One beautiful spring day I walked out of my office, twenty minutes before this patient's hour, with my appointment book lying open on my desk. I had a delicious luncheon, alone, which I enjoyed more than usual, and strolled back to the office, in time for my next appointment, only to be informed that my patient had been there and had left extremely angry. It was obvious that I had forgotten her appointment, unconsciously and purposely, and it suddenly came over me that I was absolutely fed up with her abuse to the point of nonendurance. At this point, I began to be angry at my patient, and between this time and the next time she came in, I was in a substantial rage against her. Part of this rage I related to guilt and part to some anxiety about how I would handle the next treatment interview, which I expected would surpass all previous abuse, and I was now aware of the fact that I was no longer going to be able to tolerate this abuse. I fantasied (which of course was a hope) that my patient would terminate her treatment with me. At her next appointment, she glared at me and said, in an accusatory manner, "Where were you yesterday?" I said only, "I'm sorry, I forgot." She started to attack me, saying she knew I had been there shortly before, and went on with her customary vituperation. I made no comment, for the most part feeling it was better that I say nothing. This went on for five or ten minutes and abruptly she stopped. There was a dead silence and all of a sudden she started to laugh, saying, "Well, you know, Dr. Tower, really I can't say that I blame you." This was absolutely the first break in this obstinate resistance. Following this episode, the patient was much more cooperative and after one or two short recurrences of the abusiveness, probably to test me, the defense disappeared entirely, and she shortly went into analysis at deep transference levels. At first glance, this seems so unimportant an episode that it hardly warrants description. One would say I was irritated with the patient and missed her hour because of aggression, which of course was true. But the real countertransference problem was not that. Actually, my acting-out behavior was reality-based and brought a resolution to the countertransference problem which was that I had been patient with her too long. This tendency in myself I could trace in detail from certain influences upon me in my earliest childhood. I had gotten into difficulties from this tendency from time to time during my development. I understood this in part, and yet it was not sufficiently resolved in my personality. This prolonged abusive resistance need not have lasted so long, had I been freer to be more aggressive in the face of it. The manner in which I repressed my aggression and allowed it to accumulate to a point where I was forced to act it out, was not an entirely desirable therapeutic procedure. Thus, a theoretically good therapeutic attitude, namely, that of infinite patience and effort to understand a very troubled patient, was actually in this situation a negative countertransference structure, virtually a short-lived countertransference neurosis, which undoubtedly wasted quite a bit of the patient's time, and but for my sudden resolution of it through acting out might well have gone on for a considerably longer time. I gave this little episode a good deal of thought in subsequent years, and eventually came to understand more of its true significance. (Tower, 1956, pp. 27–28)

Example 4 (from Kohut)

As I gradually began to realize, the analysand assigned to me a specific role within the framework of the world view of a very young child. During this phase of the analysis the patient had begun to remobilize an archaic, intensely cathected image of the self which had heretofore been kept in insecure repression. Concomitant with the remobilization of the grandiose self, on which she had remained fixated, there also arose the renewed need for an archaic object (a precursor of psychological structure) that would be nothing more than the embodiment of a psychological function which the patient's psyche could not yet perform for itself: to respond empathically to her narcissistic display and to provide her with narcissistic sustenance through approval, mirroring, and echoing.

Due to the fact that I was at that time not sufficiently alert to the pitfalls of such transference demands, many of my interventions interfered with the work of structure formation. But I know that the obstacles that stood in the way of my understanding lay not only in the cognitive area; and I can affirm, without transgressing the rules of decorum and without indulging in the kind of immodest self-revelation which ultimately hides more than it admits, that there were specific hindrances in my own personality which stood in the way. There was a residual insistence, related to deep and old fixation points, on seeing myself in the narcissistic center of the stage; and, although I had of course for a long time struggled with the relevant childhood delusions and thought that I had, on the whole, achieved dominance over them, I was temporarily unable to cope with the cognitive task posed by the confrontation with the reactivated grandiose self of my patient. Thus I refused to entertain the possibility that I was not an object for the patient, not an amalgam with the patient's childhood loves and hatreds, but only, as I reluctantly came to see, an impersonal function, without significance except insofar as it related to the kingdom of her own remobilized narcissistic grandeur and exhibitionism.

For a long time I insisted, therefore, that the patient's reproaches related to specific transference fantasies and wishes on the oedipal level—but I could make no headway in this direction. It was ultimately, I believe, the high-pitched tone of her voice which led me on the right track. I realized that it expressed an utter conviction of being right—the conviction of a very young child—which had heretofore never found expression. Whenever I did more (or less) than provide simple approval or confirmation in response to the patient's reports of her own discoveries, I became for her the depressive mother who (sadistically, as the patient experienced it) deflected the narcissistic cathexes from the child upon herself, or who did not provide the needed narcissistic echo. Or, I became the brother who, as she felt, twisted her thoughts and put himself into the limelight. (Kohut, 1971, pp. 287–288)

CASE REPORT: THE INNER WORLD OF A THERAPIST IN THERAPY WITH A BLIND PATIENT

The psychotherapist of a physically ill person experiences a great deal of the modal feelings evoked in ordinary interpersonal encounters with a suffering person since, even though he may understand a good deal of the underlying pathophysiology, he is not involved with the diagnosis and the therapeutics of the pathophysiology when he functions as a counselor of the self. In the case of the patient to be discussed from the point of view of the therapist, his reactions were even more intensified as the patient was a woman in her middle twenties who was blind (Ms. J. K., previously described in Chapter 4).

The therapist's initial reactions to this patient were to become caught up with the experience of sadness. At the first session, Ms. J. K. was attired in a ski-jacket and a T-shirt, which had a picture of a popular musical group, and she was at first smiling—her entire appearance was that of a pleasant and attractive young person but she carried a cane and she was obviously blind, her eyes aimlessly fixing at one point after another but never directly on the therapist's eyes or face. After she told the therapist she had asked for psychiatric help for depression, she told her story, now with appropriate affect. The essence of the patient's difficulties in her view was the lack of proper emotional support since she had become blind, which had taken place eight months ago. As previously described, the tragic circumstances were these: approximately 15 months previously, her diabetic-ridden kidneys failed and she received a kidney transplant. However, three months after this event, her poor eyesight now went completely and she became blind. At this very time, her ailing mother, who had been failing for some time, now died as yet another cerebrovascular insult hit her. Shortly after this sad event, the patient's kidney transplant began to show evidence of rejection. In the background was the history of an older brother who, four years earlier, had died in exactly the same circumstances as she now found herself—diabetic, blind, and with a uremic condition due to failing kidneys.

Her major concern focused on the inadequate attention from her father and her living brother and his wife. In her view, they did not respond appropriately to her newly experienced isolation and helplessness. She told episode after episode of their lack of accommodation to her situation. These charges seemed quite appropriate, although her father and brother, as she noted, were, over her lifetime, identified as being self-absorbed and certainly not protective towards her. Her reactions to her mother's permanent separation from her were—at least in the beginning of the therapy—sorrow for her mother's difficulties but never encompassed her own tragedy at this loss. She expressed in these sessions her lifelong experience of herself as being an inferior, a "Cinderella" person, and that each rebuff from her family served to increase her experience of herself as worthless. Her other reactions to the blindness were to make herself more self-reliant, which she attempted on many fronts—cooking, shopping, and applying for rehabilitation programs. She petitioned for psychological help when she realized her sadness was oppressive and would not remit through talking to friends and relatives and occupying herself with household duties.

After the initial experience of sorrow the therapist's inner world became filled with the familiar activity of the empathic observer, although the patient's ever-wandering eyes and her fragile appearance added to the portrait of a vulnerable and abandoned young person to whom the therapist was drawn. It was empathically clear to the therapist that his patient's physiological blindness had evoked a psychological blindness, a constriction of her experience world, a painful *aloneness*. Her experience of this constricted world was neither sufficiently altered nor relieved by people who might touch her and make her safe and comforted.

The other reactions of which the therapist became aware concerned wishes to comfort his patient through giving her desire for attention the importance he felt was indicated. The therapist understood that she needed relief from the physiological and psychological isolation in which she was mired and so, shortly after the sessions began, he gave up the usual therapeutic restraint and responded a great deal to her comments. However, the major subjective response at the beginning of the therapy was the experience of an abiding paternalistic reaction to calm, soothe, and direct the patient. This became transformed into a psychotherapeutic venture—to direct her into an unfolding and an analysis of her lifelong resistance to *receptivity*, a valid reaction to a lifelong preblindness narcissistic deprivation. As a part of her reactive fears to dependency, she had adopted a unique reaction to each human encounter: she was to be the support system; her needs for nurturance and calming were shunted aside while she became adept at keeping others in equilibrium. Along with these explorations and neutralizing of her defenses, the therapist believed that his functioning as mirror and calmer and soother would be of service in filling her self with more worth. As the sessions progressed, the patient began to experience more self-cohesion and now looked forward to going to a rehabilitation institute to which she had applied. She started her courses at this institute but her rehabilitation efforts were not to be successful. On two counts—her diabetes and her kidney failure—she began to deteriorate. The next therapy visits were after her rehabilitation work came to an end.

In the final sessions of her psychotherapy, she revealed that she was experiencing repeated hypoglycemic attacks and that her Blood Urinary Nitrogen (BUN) and Creatinine were high, signs of kidney failure. She had been on regular dialysis with frequent blood transfusions for the past year since her transplant failed; she despaired over ever getting another transplant. There was a significant change in her appearance and in her motoric behaviors; her speech and her body and facial movements were dramatically altered. Indeed, her speech was so slowed, as were her movements, as to make her unrecognizable. The dulled, sloweddown, edematous person in these sessions seemed a stranger.

In these final interviews, the patient stated that she felt hopeless that her illness would ever cease:

Therapist: What's been on your mind when you're by yourself?

Ms. J. K.: When is it all going to end? I'm so tired of being sick. It weighs on my mind. When is it going to end? It seems like everything's going bad. It's hard to wake up in the morning, there's nothing to look forward to.

Therapist: Uncertainty all the time.

Ms. J. K.: There's nothing. I don't have anyone that's real important in my life. I'm important to my dad cause I'm the link to my mom. My brother's not around. There's just not a whole lot to look forward to.

She then associated, however, to her wishes to get more relief and mentioned that she would appreciate more "effective" dialysis:

Therapist: You're certainly used to difficult and painful procedures. You're an excellent patient.

Ms. J. K.: Well, I guess I want to live. I think of my brother Steve. He just gave up. I guess I'm not ready to give up.

Therapist: You've always been able to work so well with your doctors and nurses.

Ms. J. K.: Sometimes I don't know how good I'm doing. Sometimes it begins to weigh on you.

Therapist: Tell me what you mean exactly?

Ms. J. K.: Just like, everything that happens to me—last time in the hospital, my father stayed and I felt close. He feels very sad, what did he ever do to deserve all his kids' problems? I think he feels it's his fault, it's his genes. So that's why it weighs on me.

Therapist: I think you need to be reminded that you're doing a good job. You've always done more than has been expected of you as a person and as a patient.

Ms. J. K.: What else could I do?

In this vignette, the therapy work that had been ongoing continued: the patient's need to be recognized, opposed by her pervasive fear of censure once it was expressed. In this instance the therapist attempted to support her enfeebled self, although she tried rather weakly to point to her father as the needy one.

Ms. J. K.: What should I do? Check out? Don't all people keep fighting to live?

Therapist: Even as you are in the middle of an illness, you still think of your father. You need to be reminded that you're doing a wonderful job.

Ms. J. K.: It doesn't matter how I feel, I still think of people who are close to me. Doesn't everyone?

Therapist: No. You're special in this regard. It's something to be admired.

Ms. J. K.: My grandma always tells me that. (*smile*) (*silence*) I want to thank you for helping me through everything I've been through. I really appreciate it; it's nice to know someone cares. I know it's your job but I don't think you could do it unless you really cared.

Therapist: I very much appreciate your saying that. Coming from you, that's an important comment.

Ms. J. K.: Yeah, because I really feel that if everything failed around me, I could always turn to you for support.

The psychotherapy of support enabled her to feel joined sufficiently and thus to garner the experience of being valued. The psychotherapeutic task in this situation was to attempt to continue the work of providing the requisite mirroring experiences even as she went through her by now familiar litany of her defense transference: 1) No one is around; 2) no one cares; 3) it's always been the same. These comments always served to maintain her basic defense transference posture of the "Cinderella" girl who never got the clothes or the food or the man. However, her more imminent need in the eyes of the therapist was to get a self-infusion of worth. Thus the therapist recognized her insistence that others were more needy as resistance and continued to plug into her the fuel of the mirroring functions, since she was in dire need of selfobject support.

The work-self functions as articulated in the preceding paragraphs were made difficult to implement by the shocking appearance of the patient in these final interviews: She was just not the same person. The therapist reexperienced the pathognomonic awe and inhibitions familiar to those working with hopelessly ill patients. The transference reactions in the therapist were now again observable, in this instance the uneasy entry into the experience of being with an idealized figure. In these situations the therapist became hyperreactive to the patient's expressions, especially complaints or any negative expressions which evoked *uneasiness*. It was exactly as if the therapist were in the presence of an authority figure from his past who was being severely critical, recalling the experience of ancient wishes to please. Another of the many familiar experiences for the therapist was that of the fear of being disturbing, and so if the patient indicated that she was fatigued or in pain, he was aware of the impulse to remove himself. Thus, when the patient stated, "I don't have anyone that's real important in my life . . . " and similar expressions, the *experience* of being criticized that was evoked was part of the therapist's idiosyncratic reaction to this patient, the therapist's transference.

Other manifestations of the subjective self of the therapist evident throughout the therapy were best revealed in the patient's comment at several points in the therapy: "Dr. M., you give me too many directions." She was referring to the therapist instructing her about their physical environment—how many steps to the chair or elevator, and so on. The therapist experienced from the start a strong feeling of despair in seeing this blind young woman with the ever-present smile. At different times throughout the interviews these feelings of despair became more intense, such as when the patient and the therapist would walk together and he would become more aware of his patient's helplessness. The feeling of despair was heightened during the last interview, when the patient expressed gratitude.

Does awareness of the transferences and other manifestations of the subjective self help in the handling of therapeutic encounters? This unusual activity—one might say, strange activity—of perceiving or becoming aware of one's ordinary or human self-state and its reactions and then neutralizing these reactions is a necessary and at times difficult task in performing psychotherapy. Sometimes the subjective-self reactions appear relevant to the therapeutic encounter and not idiosyncratic or part of the therapist's transference at that moment. A burst of irritation or affection or sarcasm may be experienced and even acted on and then be shrugged off as "understandable," a reaction to the patient's material or behavior that would be expected of any person to that material or behavior. The therapist is, of course, not only a "person"; the patient-therapist encounters are always to be conducted along the lines of an understanding of the patient's experiences. The patient's provocations or love-gifts are not to be hated or cherished but identified as self-experiences to be further tracked down in terms of the three phases of any therapeutic encounter: 1) the what of the experience, 2) the where-does-it-come-from; and 3) the what-is-it-doing-here now.

The intrapsychic mechanisms that are required to be in perfect operating order for the therapist to continue with his task, while being under the usual bombardment from his subjective self, are the therapist's capacity to introspect and thus "see" his subjective-self reactions, to be followed immediately by his capacities to suspend or neutralize these experiences. This latter process of isolating or walling off reactions is perhaps best thought of as a mixture of *suppression* (of behavior) and *neutralization* (of affect) and *disavowal* (a virtual self-split). The resultant self-transformation is that the therapist's self is operationally split along vertical lines. His major activity is in continuing his empathic work and therapeutic actions, while at the same time he is aware of the subjective reactions evoked by the material. The net result, when it is operational, is a manifestation of the self-forces of introspection and containment. The therapist must realize that each subjective reaction should not be discarded through justification or rationalization of one's experiences—no small task. This special "trick," to continue the work of empathically informed therapy while being barraged with *our own* reactions to competitiveness or rejections by a patient, is our greatest gift to our patients, who, if we are working well, cannot dissuade us from our goal to extricate them from their ultimately unrewarding self-states.

What does the therapist do now with these reactions? Is it enough to be vigilant and mindful of the necessity to conceive of each subjective reaction as idiosyncratic? No. The next task of the psychotherapist is that of the investigation or understanding of these subjective or transference reactions when the therapist is aware that there have been frequent episodes of their intrusion or, hopefully, when the therapist is simply making an ongoing assessment of his own transference prior to any untoward reactions. Although it is imperative that during a therapy session the therapist *become aware of* the subjective responses he is experiencing and neutralize and suppress them, he must also *study* them so as to continue to illuminate and therefore defuse the intrusive self-experiences that are always ready to interfere with his empathic work.

To return to the patient under discussion, in the reactions of the therapist to this patient suffering with blindness, diabetes, and kidney failure, there were subjective-self responses of the uneasy experience of being with an idealized figure who might become critical and express her displeasure. The therapist's reactions also included the self-experience of despair, the reaction to his patient's forced aloneness and helplessness. The study that must now be undertaken of one's revived transferences represents the therapist's continuing education. In the therapy just described with Ms. J. K. and in the therapeutic relationship with her, the revived experiences led towards an uncovering of familiar fixation points of *childhood illness* and its attendant fear of destructiveness and destructive figures, archaic complexes with which the therapist had struggled and achieved a certain dominance but had not sufficiently resolved.

Perhaps the most difficult task in becoming and being a psychotherapist lies in the work required on one's own experiences so as to make the best use of one's equipment. Reaching out to empathize, making the proper judgment about when to quietly comfort or confront—all these activities and many more require the therapist to be in optimal self-control, to know himself now and over time, so as to be able to make the least contaminated empathic diagnosis and then, on the basis of these data, perform his necessary therapeutic task.

8

An Overview:
The Clinical Theory of
Psychotherapy and the
Goals of the Psychotherapies

FLEXIBILITY IN PSYCHOTHERAPY

Although we have argued strenuously for a systematic approach to psychotherapy—the empathic diagnosis followed by a therapeutic modality with its particular technique and goals designed to alleviate the specific self-distress—we will now advance the brief that the therapist must be prepared in any of the various psychotherapy modalities to utilize *any* therapeutic technique based on the manifest problem. We are *not* advising that the overall therapeutic plan should be discarded as the material changes. Rather, we are stating our conviction that in each model of psychotherapy there will be instances in which the therapist is to use whichever techniques are of value and not be bound down by the usual techniques associated with the modality in use.

Thus, for example, it is common during an analysis for the therapist to do supportive work when his or her patient has a tragedy in the family which has evoked a painful, depressed state. The analyst in that instance will temporarily become an idealized figure who performs the task of the calmer and soother and, even,

185

advice-giver. In our experience, these intrusions into the usual work of analysis do not constitute a parameter that is harmful to the work of the analysis, especially in the work of the analysis of the transference. In any analysis extending over several years, there may be several situations during that entire timespan where the analyst is called on to reestablish intrapsychic equilibrium because of an environmental event or events that have provoked a state of intrapsychic disarray. So long as the analyst does not forget his or her place, she/he will be able to resume his or her ordinary posture as soon as there is reestablishment of self-cohesion.*

In a psychoanalytic psychotherapy, the therapist's major activity, as we have described it, is to work in alliance with the patient on significant problems which the patient is experiencing with his/her environment. However, oftentimes the therapist is called on to make interpretations of the defense transference—an activity ordinarily identified with psychoanalysis—which the patient has entered into with the therapist. This defense transference will, of course, temporarily interfere with the essential relatedness between the therapist and the patient—the therapeutic alliance. Once these interpretations of the defense transference are made and an appropriate response is forthcoming, which indicates that the patient has recognized and been able to neutralize the obstructing transference, the therapy can resume on the model of the therapist and patient examining the patient's problems with his or her environment, its people, and its institutions.

In supportive psychotherapy, there are often indications for confrontations and interpretations. These interpretations—dynamic, genetic, or transferential—are needed or even necessary in several instances. A transference interpretation is necessary when the patient is experiencing a negative transference which will interfere with the mirroring or idealized parent selfobject functions of the therapist. A dynamic interpretation—in reality, an attempt to illuminate a defense inimical to the establishment of the selfob-

---

*In his survey of 42 cases of psychoanalytic therapy, Wallerstein (1986) found that in each case of analysis supportive measures were utilized by all the analysts.

ject bond—is at times a necessary intervention. At other times, it is quite valuable to interpret to the patient a genetic pattern that enables the patient to understand and even master a defensive pattern that has been defeating to his or her self-interest, thus allowing the patient to share in the power of the idealized selfobject therapist.

In examining each of our three major therapeutic modes, we find many complexities and exceptions that emerge in the actual work of the therapies which make the notion of three discrete therapies, each with its own methodologies and goals operating for different psychopathologies, difficult to maintain. Although our goal is not, on the one hand, to maintain a rigid approach to the selection of a particular therapy for a particular self-distress, neither are we promoting the view that all therapeutic modalities work, or work as well, in all types of self-distresses. Is there a case for specificity? We will return to this query presently.

INDICATIONS, GOALS, AND METHODOLOGY IN SUPPORTIVE PSYCHOTHERAPY

In studying the indications and goals for supportive psychotherapy, it is clear that the therapist, after establishing the diagnosis of frank disarray, will best serve his/her patient by entering into the methodology identified with supportive therapy—the establishment of a self/selfobject bond which will promote psychic equilibrium. There are, as we have described, patients whose capacity for internalization is so limited that their need for a selfobject, even after equilibrium is reestablished, is more or less permanent. In these patients, whoever becomes the therapist has a selfobject function without an identifiable endpoint. We have also said about supportive therapy that the therapist must be prepared to use tools identified with other approaches when needed, such as interpretations in the face of transference behavior used in the service of restoring the therapeutic selfobject bonds. Even with all these exceptions, the therapist can be assured that there *is* a specific approach in the treatment of self-states of crisis and that the establishment of a self/selfobject bond *is* of value in self-states of fragmentation at any time in *any* therapy.

INDICATIONS, GOALS, AND METHODOLOGY IN PSYCHOANALYTIC
PSYCHOTHERAPY

Psychoanalytic psychotherapy is founded on the surmise that a limited approach to understanding a patient's self-difficulties is helpful, albeit not curative, and will bring considerable relief by causing the particular intrapsychic distress to be considerably diminished. These comments form the rationale for engaging the patient in the study of his or her particular intrapsychically formed "symptom" and actively pursuing the symptom to its genetic roots in the hope of demonstrating the past in the present.

There are instances, however, in which, even after the presenting symptom has been arrested, the self of the patient is found to have many areas of self-deficits or self-distortion which continue to erupt in new "symptoms" of difficulties with people, or at the workplace, or in his or her own continuing experience of isolation from the world. The patient's pervasive self-deficits, now more clearly apparent, require a new therapeutic diagnosis of a need for psychoanalysis. The therapist who has made the therapeutic diagnosis for psychoanalytic psychotherapy is not unaware that the "symptom" (of a work inhibition, for example) is reflective of a more global self-deficit or self-distortion. The therapeutic diagnosis of psychoanalytic psychotherapy implies that at the time of the initial diagnosis, the overall cohesiveness of the self is adequate to pursue the approach of psychotherapeutic symptom relief. Once the diagnosis changes, as it must when new or different data emerge, the therapist should have no hesitation in modifying the therapeutic approach to deal with the data of the self-distress that requires attention. This is the essence of a data-based, multi-oriented approach to psychotherapy. The following case report will describe a clinical situation that will demonstrate those situations in which the therapeutic approach required such a correction.

Case Report

Ms. E. C. came to therapy for what she referred to as "low esteem, an inability to stand up for myself" and with the painful experience of too often residing in a self of ineptitude. After it was established that she was, at this time, experiencing the symptoms of a narcissistic deficit disorder in relation to her difficulties with her fiancé, the patient was advised that psychoanalytic psychotherapy was the appropriate treatment and she started in therapy two times a week. The treatment focused on the transference she had evolved onto her fiancé, essentially a reenactment of her archaic and depriving selfobject bond with her mother. Ms. E. C. entered easily into an alliance with the therapist and did the work of therapy well; in fact, she displayed an excellent capacity for free association and for following and observing her associations. As the therapy progressed, she was able to uncover the fear of going beyond the archaic bond of childhood, the self/selfobject defense transference in which she remained the youngster, the significant other being the depriving mother. In her resistance to these insights, she developed for a brief period a defense transference to the therapist, experiencing herself as of little value and firmly believing the therapist lacked any regard for her. As the symptom of her transferential contact with her fiancé diminished, it became clear that the original therapeutic diagnosis was not to prevail, as the patient demonstrated more and more instances in other settings in which her self of ineptitude emerged. Moreover, in the therapy she began little by little to show that she was involved in thoughts and fantasies about the therapist and especially thoughts about the therapist being critical or not valuing her. After witnessing these two phenomena—the presenting symptoms disappearing and the appearance in the therapy of evidence of more extensive self-deficit—the therapist now had to undergo a shift in his version of the patient's self-cohesiveness. The patient could now be seen as a candidate for psychoanalysis.

INDICATIONS, GOALS, AND METHODOLOGY IN PSYCHOANALYSIS

In psychoanalysis, as we noted elsewhere, the psychotherapist performing the analysis must proceed with the analytic work with the assumption that the patient's self/selfobject fixations will ultimately be reactive to the analytic work and the cardinal goals of analysis—that self-growth will resume and archaic selfobject

bonds will be discarded—will be met. Of course, these are surmises and cannot be predicted prior to the analytic work. There
are instances recorded in analytic literature and in every analyst's
records in which the patient's capacity to extricate him- or herself
from the archaic bond is not sufficient to allow for growth away
from these bonds. In these instances, once the data supporting
the diagnosis of this permanent self/selfobject fixation finally become clear, the therapist is again called on to modify his/her approach and enter into a problem-solving (psychoanalytic psychotherapy) or supportive therapy mode. The following case report is
such an example.

Case Report

Ms. M. S., a 38-year-old woman, was referred for help for a
chronic depressive state and obesity. In her diagnostic interviews
she related that she was aware that her sadness and food addiction were tied up with her "real addiction—to my mother." Since
the time she had been a youngster in a family of an older and
younger brother, she was bitterly disappointed in her relationship
with her mother. Each rebuff or criticism or avoidance from her
mother would end up with the ultimate gratification of getting
contact through the contents of the refrigerator. When her mother
"woke up" to her daughter's condition when the patient was 10,
she began frantically taking her from one physician to another, to
no avail. The patient and her mother continued in combat
throughout her adolescence without any resolution of their differences. Indeed, now that she was markedly obese, all of her family
spurned her as she had become a source of embarrassment to
family and friends. Her father, a sports-minded stockbroker, was
overtly repelled by her appearance and openly avoided her in the
home.

At the end of adolescence Ms. M. S. met a sympathetic young
man bound for a career in law, and they became married when
she was 19. Through the years between the date of her marriage
and coming to see the therapist, she had worked in several different settings as typist and file clerk and finally became a real estate
broker five years prior to starting her therapy. The diagnostic data

revealed a highly intelligent woman who suffered with episodes of total self-bankruptcy, during which times she could not arise from her bed. Her relationship with her husband was cordial but unfulfilling. He was one of those men driven to achieve monetary success and who, therefore, spent each working hour on money-making schemes. The symptom of compulsive eating, especially the night-eating syndrome, had waned for a few years directly after the marriage but was again dominating her life. The eating now began with little in the way of overt or recognized psychological stimuli, although Ms. M.S. still had violent reactions to her mother's daily phone calls. These reactions consisted of severe anxiety during her mother's call, followed almost immediately by rushing to the refrigerator for anything to "fill me up." She still had a repetitious dream—a nightmare—in which she found herself *inside* a huge refrigerator attempting unsuccessfully to grab frantically at all and any of the food contents within the refrigerator. She demonstrated an adequate capacity for self-awareness with little or no uneasiness to the therapist's confrontations. It was decided to start her in four-times-a-week analysis.

The first phase of her analysis found her able to report her inner life without tension and to join in an exploration of deeper mental contents. However, shortly after this interlude she began centering her comments on her mother and husband; they were, of course, interchangeable. These comments were all filled with her list of disappointments in their inability to attend to her. Her mother and husband were too busy so that their ministrations were never able to satiate her. Before long, the therapist was added to the list, and now in the analysis she complained that the therapist was too busy and too distracted or too involved in others to attend to her. The interpretations given to her were not used by her to study her self-state. During these experiences of deprivation, she experienced the therapist's comments as if he were simply demeaning her. As this phase continued (by now, the patient had been in analysis for 15 months), it became clear that either the patient was in an intractable defense transference or the defense transference phase of analysis would be lengthy since it was so pervasive and intense. Nine months afterwards, the analyst continued to wait it out and offer defense transference interpretations but, as it turned out, to no avail. The patient continued "being" in 1953, not in 1983.

This is a case of an archaic and adhesive self/selfobject bond which is so often refractory to any psychotherapeutic ministrations. The patient unconsciously insisted on living as a deprived youngster and fighting off all challenges to the archaic bonds, which she continued to reenact in all human encounters. Her attachments to her mother were experienced by her as necessary for survival. Whomever she encountered became her mother, who *is* the purveyor of life. Thus her capacity to bond with the therapist as therapist to patient was limited, as was her overall capacity to remove herself from the self of the chronically underfed youngster in contact with the current selfobject mother. In effect, she returned to the self-of-inferiority and depletion several times a day. This world of being the underfed youngster was her *only* source of security—love, direction, and guidance. She had always associated assertiveness and the success that went with it with "terminal aloneness"; love and togetherness were associated with the youngster who needed protection in a merger with a selfobject mother.

The previously established therapeutic diagnosis, therefore, was not valid; the patient *could not* free herself from the malignant transference without experiencing a disintegration anxiety. The analyst was called on now to modify the therapy in accord with the data and conclude that the patient would best be served by supportive psychotherapy, i.e., that the therapist must *"be"* an archaic selfobject and perform the functions of the idealized parent imago. Could this patient's intractable adhesiveness to her archaic selfobjects have been diagnosed earlier? Perhaps the most informed view is that the diagnosis of treatability requires a test of treatment so that the treatment process requires constant evaluation.

ON THE NECESSITY OF AN ONGOING ASSESSMENT IN PSYCHOTHERAPY

Thus, while the motto for one diagnosis means that one therapeutic approach should continue to be the prevailing theme for psychotherapists, the therapist is to be mindful of perhaps a more important principle: Our therapies are to be relevant to the data we have gathered. As Freud (1913) taught long ago, each therapy case is on probation during its initial life. Our view is that it is necessary to extend this period of probation throughout the therapy so that the therapist continues his observations about the worthwhileness of his therapeutic plan until he is assured that the therapeutic modality in use is the proper therapeutic approach and that the therapy is proceeding well. The answer to our query about the case for specificity then becomes that there *is* a case for specificity of goals and methodologies in psychotherapy but that these goals are subject to change should the self-needs of the patient become altered. At any stage of the therapy, the therapist must be receptive to the need for a change in the therapy.

Stepping back from the details of the work performed in psychotherapy of any type, the therapist will find it helpful to review from time to time the self-development of the individual under his charge. The object of our study is to put in place once again the self of the patient and his capacities for mutual studying and the capacity to invest in an object other than the archaic selfobject and self-functions. A key word here is *capacity*, implying that in the future the functions observed, e.g., the self-observing function, may be capable of growth.

For example, the *theory and practice of psychotherapy* are based on the notion that a bond formed between the patient and his/her therapist can be used to alleviate psychic distress through archaic nurturance (supportive therapy), or reexamining a sector of one's past (psychoanalytic psychotherapy), or reliving and thus studying this reliving (psychoanalysis). These bonds utilized for therapeutic purposes are essentially transferences, and all psychotherapies reflect the differential workings of the transference in terms of what uses are made of the transference, from support to analysis.

We always start and end our clinical encounters with the data of the presenting self. For example, our first patient may have a self in distress but not in disarray; his cognitive functions are all intact; his anxiety has not invaded his thinking processes. Our next subject presenting for psychotherapy is in a state of fragmentation; either her grief has overwhelmed her or her anxiety has become panic, and she cannot function at this moment since her thinking and perceptions are derailed. Our next investigations, after these self-diagnoses, will turn to the *self-functions* present and our surmises about their potential for growth or usage in the therapy. Each of the approaches to psychotherapy—support, problem-solving, psychoanalysis—has a psychic-tool requirement. In supportive therapy the requirements are more modest than those for problem-solving therapy, but they are necessary. To gain relief through supportive therapy requires that the subject's distress not be overwhelming so that language and nonverbal attitudes can be utilized.

In those therapies that will ultimately involve self-observation, the therapist has to judge the present or potential capacity for insight, knowing that in the midst of a transference experience, this self-function will be affected and temporarily paralyzed so that these diagnoses are only provisional but important to ascertain. Without the evidence that the patient can utilize insight to some extent, the therapist cannot go forward in prescribing psychoanalytic therapy or psychoanalysis. There can never be a formation of an alliance, a mutual studying, without this self-function being operational.

The therapist in those clinical situations in which psychoanalytic therapy or psychoanalysis will be used must judge the patient's capacity for transference and to make a judgment of whether or not the transference will be "workable," capable of a resolution, or conversely will never be capable of resolution and become transformed into a deterrent to the progress of the therapy. As previously noted, a good deal of these data can only be gleaned during the course of the therapy—for example, the data of the so-called "workable transference." Some of these data can be recognized from the patient's history of his or her object and selfobject relationships.

Perhaps the most difficult assessment to make in our work is in the area at times referred to as the patient's capacity for change, the depth of fixations, and so on. There are those patients who seemingly are not capable of investing in a bond with a therapist in any manner; they are functionally unable to bond with anyone other than their archaic selfobject. In these persons one can say

they are incapable of change, although at what point in the therapy would this assessment be finally valid? The therapy or analysis
would have to proceed for a considerable period before a therapist
would, or should, feel that the diagnosis of unchangeability is
valid. Fixations—their nature, their genesis, their mutability—are
what psychotherapy is all about since they are one of the most
important elements in psychopathology. In a sense, all psychotherapists devote a good deal of their thought and effort over their
lifetimes to an understanding of their patients' fixations. Other
patients who are capable of forming a transference and experience
need and disappointment and bonding to their therapist will yet
have massive resistance to the final extrication from their fixations
when it comes to the ultimate separations—in the transference
and in their outer world of objects and selfobjects. We are here
speaking of fixations of their archaic self/selfobject encounters so
that, for example, the spouse who had formerly been experienced
as an archaic selfobject will no longer be experienced in psychotherapy or psychoanalysis as the tyrant with whom the patient
maintains an archaic bond. At times one can form an appreciation
for the depth of the fixations from the history of object and selfobject relationships in which it becomes clear that the patient, while
seemingly involved in many human encounters, in actuality reveals a sameness in his/her selfobject bonds, still attempting to
extricate from his/her current selfobject what was missing in the
way of nurturance or control or direction or calming–soothing.

In other clinical encounters, the therapy may move along well
for considerable time until it is clear that a plateau of understanding or movement has been reached. And then in response to the
need for a major alteration or a reaction to an event in the patient's
life, it is revealed that the patient turns back to archaic gratification
or has never been fully removed from these archaic sources of
direction. The importance of assaying and continuing to assay the
fixations present in the patient and the capacity for change or
movement or growth is that it defines the type of therapy possible
and defines the time requirements for the resolution of the self-
difficulty which, at times, will simply be stated as "cannot be
determined."

Now we are at the stage of appreciation of the uniqueness and similar features of our therapeutic approaches based on our data of:

1) the presenting self-state (functions in operation; inoperative functions);
2) the dominant self-needs (current and characterological);
3) the patient's self-development, with a special emphasis on the history of selfobject and self/selfobject relationships;
4) the self-functions required for the recommended therapy;
5) the goals of the therapy;
6) the course of the therapy and the capacity for termination.

As we have indicated in this chapter and elsewhere in this volume, in each clinical instance in which the patient requires an alteration in the therapeutic plan, the maxim must be that it is the empathically derived data that dictate the therapeutic approach. From the clinical theory viewpoint, it is the self/selfobject need at the moment that will dictate the therapeutic posture. In those selves—regardless of the previously prescribed plan—who become immersed in a state of disarray, the self-need is for calming and soothing. The appropriate methodology is to enlist a selfobject presence to help in the formation of a self/selfobject bond. And, as we have already indicated, in those instances in which the prescribed therapy has been the supportive approach, the therapist has commonly to utilize the methodology of the psychoanalytic approaches—confrontation, interpretations of all kinds, abstinence, and so on. The psychoanalytic approaches in these instances are derived from the empathically derived awareness that there is resistance to forming the self/selfobject bond necessary to obtain relief from the self-distress.

In each of the self-states of distress, the therapist will be monitoring the progress throughout the therapy to evaluate whether or not the therapy continues to be relevant for the patient or whether the patient requires alteration in frequency of visits, more or less in the way of intervention (interpretation, confrontation), or whether the patient would be better helped by another approach.

Our approach to psychotherapy should always be based on the

minute-to-minute empathic survey of the self-state of our patients and, from this scrutiny, to plug in what is required. In a specific clinical instance, the attention is to maintain the equilibrium; in another instance, to further the self-growth away from the patient's constant structuring of archaic mirroring self/selfobject encounters which constantly stifles his or her growth in becoming a creative, assertive person.

ON ALTERING THE THERAPEUTIC MODALITY

The following two reports are presented to demonstrate the intricacies encountered at times in the practice of psychotherapy, especially in the realm of the changing self-need and the necessity to be vigilant about altering the therapeutic modality in response to the changing self-need.

Case 1

Mr. J. C., a 36-year-old single accountant who lived with his mother, came to therapy for treatment of a depression which started, in his view, from overwork and not enough attention to his bodily needs. He had been transferred to another city as part of a promotion in his accounting firm, a large national organization. Three or four months after this transfer, he developed a persistent insomnia and, coupled with his now-present anorexia, he lost a considerable amount of weight in a few weeks. Troubled by these events, he became despondent and asked to be returned home for medical treatment. His internist, noting his dysphoria as well as his psychomotor retardation, referred him for treatment of what seemed to be a depressive state. In his diagnostic interview, Mr. J. C. stated that the transfer from his hometown was part of a wish on his part to move away from his mother and was actually the first separation from her in his adult life. In fact, as he related, he had never become intimate with anyone over time nor was there a woman in his life. He had had some chums who accompanied him to school but as soon as school was over, he usually ran home. This pattern persisted throughout grammar school and high school. In college he went to a local university so that each weekend he was again with his mother. There were no interferences from the rest of the family into his life or his mother's life. His father had died when he was three in an industrial accident. After this event, he was told, his mother became despondent and, although she was quite attractive and young, she never dated again. She took a job at a nearby school as a typist so that she would be close to her growing child and devoted her life to his development.

His mother's unique influence on him became apparent from the earliest of his days. She rewarded quietness, studiousness, and gentleness and totally rejected rowdyism and athletics. She would take the patient into her bed each night, he remembered, and read him poetry and passages from the Bible, mythology, and stories from the *Reader's Digest*. Later on, in each grade of grammar school, he remembered that his mother was involved in each of his schoolwork assignments. He also recalled that she was critical of any chums he might bring home, usually because of their manners or rowdiness. She would often tell him, as he grew older, to be cautious about getting involved with girls as they would only be interested in "tying him down" so that he would never finish his education. Once, on the occasion of a high school dance, he brought home his date for the evening. His mother apparently stayed in her room and refused to meet his date. For the next week, she hardly spoke to him and refused to eat meals with him. When she finally broke her silence, it was to remind him, over and over again, about the pitfalls of getting involved with women. He found himself so distressed by his mother's withdrawal that he resolved never to bring home another woman. After the one or two high school dances he attended, he did not date again for the next 20 years to the time he came for therapy. He said in his diagnostic session that the reaction from his mother should he go out on a date would "not be worth it," indicating that his anxiety at the prospect of her disapproval would be overwhelming and impossible to tolerate.

He had viewed his transfer to another city as a passageway to freedom which he himself could not initiate; but under the guise of a commanded transfer, he could leave his mother with impunity. It was clear to him in his new assignment that he had become more and more uneasy away from his mother, even a little paranoid at the prospect that she was following him. Actually, when work ended he raced home fearful that she might call and that he would not be home to receive the call; thus he would open himself up for criticism from her for again being too interested in playful activities or eating with women. When he left his out-of-town assignment, he resumed living with his mother.

Mr. J. C.'s first self-need was to be calmed in a supportive psychotherapy setting, as he revealed an agitated state in his first encounters with the therapist. After only a few diagnostic visits the therapist saw him every other day and instructed him to arrange for an indefinite medical leave of absence. The initial visits were confined to instructing him how to spend the day since he was not able to communicate a great deal. He was told how much to sleep, how much activity he should try to have, and how much rest during the day. He was told to make a plan for each segment of the day or each hour so that there would be little unstructured time. He was also advised about what shows to watch on television. Although he was told that the therapist would speak to his mother, she never called. The therapist continued for four weeks to see him every other day, and he began to tell of the historical events outlined above, especially centering on his relationship with his mother. After five weeks, the patient and therapist decided he would start back at work, at first part-time. At the beginning of his problem, the patient had gone to see an internist in the town he was in and was judged to be without metabolic disease or gastrointestinal abnormalities.

After a few more months Mr. J. C. reported that his vigor had returned as had his appetite, and his insomnia and early morning arising had disappeared. In the therapy sessions, now three times a week, the therapist and patient discussed a variety of topics centered on Mr. J. C.'s interests—none that he ever ventured into if it involved leaving his home. He knew a great deal about athletics of all kinds; he kept up quite well with current events and he was a reader of books, novels, and mysteries. He mentioned that his involvement with his mother for the past decade or more was only that they took meals together and that they watched some TV shows together. But, he stated, they passed only one or two words to each other all evening; even during dinner they rarely spoke. She had stopped inquiring about his life at the office. On a rare occasion when he left the house after dinner, she did not question him as to his whereabouts. They, in effect, were not in contact after dinner and, as noted, during dinner there was rarely a word passed between them. The pattern of his week now became clear; he went to work each day, returning home almost precisely at the same time each evening. After his evening return to his home, he did not go out again. Weekends, without the required trip to the office, he spent entirely in his home with his mother. The evening and weekend were spent in a state of isolation with the TV and books from time to time. No relatives had called for years; his mother did *no* socializing.

In the third month of his therapeutic work, the investigation into Mr. J. C.'s personal life began with the therapist staking out an area for psychoanalytic psychotherapy. The supportive therapy had resulted in the patient's experiencing a return of his self-cohesiveness. He, in fact, proclaimed that he "felt better" than he had ever felt in his life. It now seemed clear that an attempt should be made to investigate this intense self/selfobject fixation in a man who was intelligent, who related with keen awareness (insight) that he felt uneasy in leaving the bondage with his mother, and who wished to dissolve the bonds of imprisonment. In fact, shortly after the therapy began to focus on the imprisonment of his self, he began to run each morning for increasing distances (8–10 miles). This was also a sign that he could move from the selfobject binding. He quickly understood the archaic imprisoning selfobject bonds and the transferential aspects of this binding—his mother had displayed very little interest in his extra-work activities over the past decade.

Months passed by and the patient continued to feel well but the therapy sessions became a monotonous succession of discussing weekly events, from current events to athletics, and then centering again and again on the single proposition—the confrontation that he was uneasy over his mother's negative responses to any sign of his leaving home for leisure or social activities. He agreed with this proposition but then was unable to elaborate further with an exposition of his reactions to his mother's covert commands to remain a prisoner at home. He also began to report, now six months later, that he suddenly became lethargic on Saturday afternoons when he began to make plans to go to the movies or any of the local restaurants. Now, towards the end of the first year, each visit (they were now two times a week at his request, the patient complaining of the inordinate amount of time required to meet with the therapist) was so stereotyped that one could predict when the therapist would confront him about his inability to leave the house once again. Mr. J. C. would plead laziness or apathy or embarrassment about going without a companion to a restaurant or movie house. He remained unreactive to the proposition (confrontation) that he and the therapist were, once again, looking at the exhibition of a youngster frightened to desperation, although he agreed that he was certainly immobilized and that he certainly carried around a great deal of respect for his mother that was unwarranted. After one-and-a-half years of attempting to form an alliance of goals so that he, with his therapist, could study the major pathological sector of his self, there had been little progress.

This case represents an instance in which the patient's *capacity* to form an alliance was so minimal at first that it was not up to the work of psychoanalytic psychotherapy. The patient's capacity to invest in any other relationship save his contact with his mother was almost nonexistent. He was frightened to form a relationship with anyone lest his mother know of it. The transference onto his mother as *the* only supplier of his worth, the supplier of oxygen, dominated his life and, above all, could never be challenged or in any way diluted lest his mother hear of it and then punish him, ultimately to desert him.

Forming an alliance with another person and self-observing are psychic operations that reflect the experience of safety in moving away from childhood selfobjects into introspection and dialogue with another. Conversely, in self/selfobject encounters in childhood in which the selfobject is *not* experienced as a consistent mirroring presence, the child does not move away freely but actually is *rooted* to the ancient relationship in the same self-posture of childhood—too frightened to move or even move his or her eyes from the selfobject since there is no *assurance*, through her constant mirroring presence, that she will continue to be there regardless of what the child's behavior will be or with whom the child interacts.

Mr. J. C. continued to listen politely to the therapist's confrontation, which stressed that he was living in an archaic world, essentially in a defense transference, with continuing fear of his mother's abandonment if he ventured out of her field of vision. The problem was that he could not sufficiently ally himself with the therapist nor could he observe this unique childhood self in operation since he was, or *became*, each day he went home, the youngster. He was totally immersed in the fixation of his childhood defense transference as his mature self-functions, such as self-observing, were not operational. The therapist was, in fact, for a long time talking to a child, although he had the outward appearance of an attractive, sober-minded and sober-looking, tall and aesthetic man.

Mr. J. C. said to the therapist during that long period in his therapy when he was immobilized, "I just can't get myself to move out of that home; there's no one around to stop me. She's not even around when I should be going out on Saturday or on week nights. I just can't get mobilized. I don't have any rationalization to use; I just can't get mobilized." The therapist struggled to empathize with that experience since it was difficult to capture that immobilizing fear of a mother's withdrawal. It is important to note here that this was a crucial event in the therapy since once the therapist could make that empathic leap and appreciate the depth and tenacity of the fixation, he would be more tenacious in pursuing the careful and persistent work required in this psychotherapy. The therapist's task was to help this man feel the positive and safe ambience of his therapeutic relationship so that he could maintain a tie with the therapist and the therapist's functions, especially in self-observing—in"seeing" himself enter into the regressive self/selfobject status of childhood in which he could not remove himself from his mother's presence—frozen like a statue in her field of vision.

After some 14 months had elapsed, the patient began to show changes in his behavior, especially at work, in his ability to interact with his colleagues and his own staff. His presentations at work in front of small groups became easier and he even received compliments for this activity. He reported to the therapist that he had started conversations with several women at his age level in his firm and considered going to lunch with one of them in the future. He also reported that he was feeling more vigor than ever before. In the therapy, however, he continued to be a minimal participant in his responsiveness to the defense transference interpretations. He has not yet demonstrated that he can consistently "see" himself entering into the world of 1953 where he had to submerge his self to survive. However, he has demonstrated significant behavioral change and certainly feels an enhanced self. This therapy is ongoing and will be for an extended time.

This case record demonstrates a complex problem in the practice of psychotherapy. The initial empathic diagnosis of a self-state of a painful depression was clear, and the therapeutic diagnosis of supportive psychotherapy was likewise clear. Indeed, Mr. J. C. did respond to the therapeutic ministrations of the selfobject functioning of the therapist and regained his self-cohesion. After he was restored to his premorbid self, it became evident that he was unconsciously living in a prison of psychic deprivation—a reenactment of his lonely, empty childhood, salvaged only by the reassurance that his mother would be stationary so long as he retained the posture of the passive and obedient son. He was, of course, aware only of the empty, lonely experiences for which he wished relief and, later, of the absolute impossibility, or so it seemed, of leaving "her" house. The problem that this distorted self presented was that in order to move from his position on his developmental ladder, he must become aware of his continual reentry into the archaic self/selfobject dyad of his childhood. This awareness, this problem solving of the pathological sector, requires the tools of self-observing and the ability to form an alliance, basically an offshoot of the alter ego twinship transference. Our patient, as we have described, at the time of his entry into psychotherapy did not show that he had these qualifications; however, his self-state of misery, based as it is on the reenactment of his malignant self/selfobject dyad of childhood, will not vanish of its own volition. In these situations, the therapist is compelled to engage in this long-term project in an attempt to salvage this patient, armed as he is with the empathically derived knowledge that he will be in combat with a tenaciously fixated self over an extended period of time.

Case 2

Ms. M. F., a 34-year-old married woman, mother of two children, presented for therapy self-referred since she was aware that she was in a chronically agitated and depressed state and that she was becoming addicted to the use of amphetamines to alleviate her "down periods," as she referred to them. Her self-state was clear: she was experiencing periods of self-fragmentation whenever her self-needs were intense. She was in need of calming and soothing *now*. The therapy plan was to engage in supportive work, which was started immediately. She was seen frequently during this time with attention paid to regulating her home life which had become so chaotic, with no set times for any of the usual domestic duties or childrearing functions. She was also put on a schedule for the amphetamines she was using in a random pattern and, later on, she began to decelerate the use of these compounds. After about three months of this combination of functioning as the idealized parent who directs and calms and regulates and as the mirroring selfobject who places the youngster on stage center, she did become more cohesive.

Now that her cohesive self was reestablished, it became apparent that she was involved in a marriage which was, for her, a reliving of being the unwanted daughter of a hostile and ungrateful mother—in this instance, often replaying this scene with a husband who was neither hostile nor ungrateful but who was unaware of her psychic structuring of their relationship. Indeed, he did not know what hit him when, several times a week (some-times every night during a particular week) she would explode with accusations about his lack of regard or his disrespect or his interest in other women at his laboratory. He was a biologist in a pharmaceutical company and was, from her many consistent de-scriptions, a good person and a devoted husband and father to their three- and six-year-old daughters. These episodes of feeling inept in relating to her husband and daughters had started in earnest after the first pregnancy and increased markedly after the second child was born. At that time they moved away from their home and families in the East to the midwest, where her husband had been offered a highly important job. In Ms. M. F.'s back-ground stood a special relationship with a chronically ill mother and an older sister, who was the operational mother in the family.

It seemed to this patient that from her earliest days, she used to tiptoe around her mother lest her mother launch into an attack on her for being inconsiderate to an ill and "dying" person. Her mother was apparently confined to her bed for considerable time with a variety of maladies: congestive heart failure, asthma, arthropathy, and anemia of unknown origin. The patient was placed under the leadership of her older sister to whom she al-ways felt inferior and of whom she was frightened, since she was given to lashing out at Ms. M. F. with whatever she had in her hand, including her fists, for minor infractions. She always re-membered her father as the "nice guy" in the house but who also joined the family game plan of maintaining the mother's equilibri-um through quietness and frequent gestures of pity and obedi-ence to her whims. In this milieu the patient learned to suppress her wants and to run to others for help. She remembered running away from home since she was a toddler and always being found by her father who, in her view, was made by others in the family to spank her. These escapades stopped when she was seven or eight years old when her mother was carried away to the hospital for another episode of heart trouble. On this occasion, her sister accused her of causing mother's difficulties and, as Ms. M. F. remembered it 25 years later, told her that her mother would die because of her running away. This patient apparently underwent a personality change in her early teens, becoming a meek, unobtrusive, and accommodating youngster who was good in school and as a domestic at home, learning to cook and clean in an expert manner. She raced through college and graduate school, where she met her husband, and earned a master's degree in microbiology.

Until the first pregnancy, she and her husband apparently lived well with one another. Almost in tandem with the pregnancy, the patient underwent a self-transformation in the direction of episodes of low self-regard and paranoid accusations against her husband. She had a return of her old behavior of "running away," this time for hours, even overnight, sleeping in the family car. After the pregnancy, she again resumed her previous accommodating behavior, nursed her firstborn, and was pleasant for the most part at home with her husband. When she decided to become pregnant again, it was with the expectation that she would be fine. However, again with the pregnancy came the regressive appearance of the inferior-feeling, angered person looking for a fight. This pregnancy was even more tumultuous in terms of the multiple episodes of disarray and violent behavior and incidences of running away.

After this pregnancy, Ms. M. F. developed a more malignant symptom than her previous ones: she started using amphetamine capsules which she had used at other times for weight control and for examination fatigue during graduate school. However, she used them as much as five to six times more than had been prescribed and, at times, was clearly hypomanic in her behavior, with frequent outbursts of agitated, angry behavior and anorexia and sleeplessness. The self-state diagnosis was clear now, as well as the self-need for an understanding and problem solving of the return of the Cinderella-self into her psyche. The therapeutic strategy now was to isolate for her the current central lesion: the reliving of the unimportant little girl attempting to gain acceptance from her selfobject, now experienced as her husband in the transference. Here is another instance of the therapist's need to alter his therapeutic strategy to match the new self-need. In the case of Ms. M. F., psychoanalytic psychotherapy had to be instituted at this juncture.

In this complicated, regressive self-state, Ms. M. F. became the shabby little girl whose selfobject mother would demean and utter vituperations at her. The little girl would have to run away to get help or, as in this case, use amphetamines to help remove the state of shabbiness. Her husband, in the role assigned to him in this unconscious drama, would be hateful to her, invested in another woman. Our patient would attempt to replay this drama often during the week, insisting that her husband "must" conceive of her as the little "retard" who was greedy and unsympathetic— exactly what her mother used in railing at her.

In a nutshell, the patient responded to the therapist's intervention of confronting her with the insistence on her part that her husband had to relive with her the tragic scenes of her childhood. Her need to be with mother in the old way, that of being the demeaned youngster genuflecting to her monarch, revealed that her ancient fixation, the only way to garner some degree of nurturance, was again holding sway over her self. She needed to "see" this revisitation of her former self/selfobject dyad as yet another attempt to gain love from her mother-husband—of course, in the only way possible for her as the ugly duckling. Once she could see this reliving and separate from the reflexly induced self of ineptitude, she could enter into the camaraderie and warmth of her marriage. Indeed, she did, over the next many months (although with many episodes of running away and with amphetamines) begin to dissect out those episodes of the emerging little girl self in which she would attempt to revisit with her husband those childhood scenes of depreciation.

The patient entered into a defense transference with the therapist on several occasions and sometimes for protracted periods. During these times the total immersion of the self into a violent paranoid person was impressive, as was her resistance to working on the eruption of this self and the self/selfobject complex in the therapy. On the whole the most important ingredient in the resolution of the defense transference was the increasing awareness on her part of her need to reinstitute with the therapist the ancient forces of equilibrium, she being the subjugated servant begging for oppression and the therapist being the tyrant. Once this dyad was recognized, no matter what the extent of the provocation, the therapist could continue with his goal to get the patient to "see" the malignant dyad instituted vis-à-vis her husband. On several occasions the patient articulated this by stating: "I've tried many times to get kicked out of here or get you to fight like I want my husband to, but I never win! I think that helped me get over this crap!"

After four-and-a-half years the patient and the therapist terminated her treatment. She had come in several times over the succeeding eight years to discuss situations in which she wanted advice or direction. One episode resulted in her seeing the therapist for four consecutive weeks.

This last case illustrates, among other things, the therapeutic results possible when the fixations are not as adhesive as in other clinical situations. This patient could join with the therapist (although after the working out of the defense transference to the therapist) and develop insight into her malignant self of childhood. In an attempt to understand what was there in her depriving background that did not cause her to become permanently fixated on inferiority and refractory to change, we can list the following variables: 1) Ms. M. F. was successful in her roles of student and scientist; 2) she did experience love with and from her husband, indicating some connection unknown to the therapist between appreciation and love in her childhood; 3) her very early years (first 24 months) may have been somewhat positive since she was, and is, an emotionally wise and engaging person— perhaps as a result of having been cuddled and caressed and cherished.

Perhaps the most important learning that comes from this and other clinical experiences is that the therapist must initiate each case as a researcher. Each clinical encounter should be undertaken with the attitude of experimentation, since in our field we cannot predict the extent and depth of the resistance to change which is the single most important ingredient in the success or failure of our therapies. Therefore, the therapist must begin each clinical encounter as an investigator. The voyage of psychotherapy cannot be charted in advance.

Bibliography

Alexander, F. (1963). The dynamics of psychotherapy in the light of learning theory. *American Journal of Psychiatry, 120,* 440–448.

Alexander, F., & French, T. (1946). *Psychoanalytic therapy: Principles and applications.* New York:The Ronald Press Company.

Arlow, J. A. (1963). The supervisory situation. *Journal of the American Psychoanalytic Association, 11,* 576–594.

Bacal, H. A. (1985). Optimal responsiveness and the therapeutic process. In A. Goldberg (Ed.), *Progress in self psychology* (vol. 1, pp. 202–227). New York: Guilford Press.

Balint, M. (1968). *The basic fault: Therapeutic aspects of regression.* London: Tavistock.

Basch, M. F. (1980). *Doing psychotherapy.* New York: Basic Books.

Basch, M. F. (1981). Selfobject disorders and psychoanalytic theory: A historical perspective. *Journal of the American Psychoanalytic Association, 29,* 337–351.

Basch, M. F. (1983a). Empathic understanding: A review of the concept and some theoretical considerations. *Journal of the American Psychoanalytic Association, 31,* 101–126.

Basch, M. F. (1983b). Affect and the analyst. *Psychoanalytic Inquiry, 3,* 691–703.

Basch, M. F. (1983c). The significance of self psychology for a theory of psychotherapy. In J. Lichtenberg & S. Kaplan (Eds.), *Reflections in self psychology.* New York: International Universities Press.

Basch, M. F. (1984a). Selfobjects, development and psychotherapy. In P. Stepansky & A. Goldberg (Eds.), *Kohut's legacy: Contributions to self psychology.* Hillsdale, NJ: Analytic Press.

Basch, M. F. (1984b). Selfobjects and selfobject transference: Theoretical implications. In P. E. Stepansky & A. Goldberg (Eds.), *Kohut's legacy: Contributions to self psychology.* Hillsdale, NJ: Analytic Press.

Brandschaft, B. & Stolorow R. (1984). Borderline concept: Pathological character or iatrogenic myth? In J. Lichtenberg, M. Burnstein, & D. Silver (Eds.), *Empathy II.* Hillsdale, NJ: The Analytic Press.

Daniels, R. (1976). Manifestations of transference: Their implication for the first phase of psychoanalysis. *Journal of the American Psychoanalytic Association, 17,* 995–1014.

Deutsch, F. (1949). *Applied psychoanalysis: Selected objectives of psychotherapy*. New York: Grune & Stratton.

Dewald, P. (1964). *Psychotherapy: A Dynamic approach*. New York: Basic Books.

Dewald, P. (1972). *The psychoanalytic process*. New York: Basic Books.

Dostoyevsky, F. (1878). *Notes from underground*. New York: New American Library, 1961.

Fenichel, O. (1941). *Problems of psychoanalytic technique*. Albany, NY: The Psychoanalytic Quarterly.

Ferenczi, S., & Rank, O. (1925). *The development of psychoanalysis*. New York: Nervous and Mental Disease Publishing Company.

Fliess, R. (1942). The metapsychology of the analyst. *Psychoanalytic Quarterly, 11*, 211-227.

Freud, S. (1912a). The dynamics of transference. *Standard Edition, 12*, 97108. London: Hogarth Press, 1958.

Freud, S. (1912b). Recommendations to physicians practising psychoanalysis. *Standard Edition, 12*. London: Hogarth Press, 1958.

Freud, S. (1913). On beginning the treatment. *Standard Edition, 12*, 121-144. London: Hogarth Press, 1958.

Freud, S. (1914). Remembering, repeating and working through. *Standard Edition, 12*, 145-157. London: Hogarth Press, 1958.

Freud, S. (1915). Observations on transference-love. *Standard Edition, 12*, 157-172. London: Hogarth Press, 1958.

Freud, S. (1917a). Mourning and melancholia. *Standard Edition, 14*, 237-259. London: Hogarth Press, 1958.

Freud, S. (1917b). Introductory lectures on psycho-analysis. Part III, Lecture XXVII, Transference. *Standard Edition, 16*, 431-447. London: Hogarth Press, 1963.

Freud, S. (1917c). Introductory lectures on psycho-analysis. Part III, Lecture XXVIII, Analytic therapy. *Standard Edition, 16*, 448-463. London: Hogarth Press, 1963.

Freud, S. (1921). Group psychology and the analysis of the ego. *Standard Edition, 18*, 65-144. London: Hogarth Press, 1958.

Freud, S. (1926). Inhibitions, symptoms and anxiety. *Standard Edition, 20*, 75-174. London: Hogarth Press, 1958.

Freud, S. (1937). Analysis terminable and interminable. *Standard Edition, 22*, 209-255. London: Hogarth Press, 1958.

Gedo, J., & Goldberg, A. (1973). *Models of the mind: A psychoanalytic theory*. Chicago: University of Chicago Press.

Gill, M. M. (1954). Psychoanalysis and exploratory psychotherapy. *Journal of the American Psychoanalytic Association, 2*, 771-797.

Gitelson, M. (1952). The emotional position of the analyst in the psychoanalytic situation. *International Journal of Psycho-Analysis, 33*, 1-10.

Gitelson, M. (1962. The curative factor in psychoanalysis: The first phase of psychoanalysis intervention. *International Journal of Psycho-Analysis, 43*, 194-234.

Glover, E. (1928). *The technique of psychoanalysis*. London: Baillière, Tindal, & Cox.

Goldberg, A. (1975). Narcissism and the readiness for psychotherapy termination. *Archives of General Psychiatry, 29*, 695-704.

Goldberg, A. (Ed.) (1978). *Psychology of the self: A casebook*. New York: International Universities Press.

Goldberg, A. (Ed.) (1980). *Advances in self psychology*. New York: International Universities Press.

Goldberg, A. (Ed.) (1983). *The future of psychoanalysis*. New York: International Universities Press.

Greenson, R. (1958). The working alliance and the transference neurosis. *Psychoanalytic Quarterly, 34*, 155–181.

Greenson, R. (1967). *The technique and practice of psychoanalysis. Vol. 1*. New York: International Universities Press.

Greenson, R., & Wexler, M. (1969). The non-transference relationship in the psychoanalytic situation. *International Journal of Psycho-Analysis, 50*, 27–39.

Kohut, H. (1959). Introspection, empathy and psychoanalysis. *Journal of the American Psychoanalytic Association, 7*, 459–483.

Kohut, H. (1966). Forms and transformations of narcissism. *Journal of the American Psychoanalytic Association, 14*, 243–273.

Kohut, H. (1968). The psychoanalytic treatment of narcissistic personality disorders: Outline of a systematic approach. *The Psychoanalytic Study of the Child, 23*, 86–114.

Kohut, H. (1971). *Analysis of the self*. New York: International Universities Press.

Kohut, H. (1972). Thoughts on narcissism and narcissistic rage. *The Psychoanalytic Study of the Child, 27*, 360–400.

Kohut, H. (1974). Remarks about the formation of the self. In P. Ornstein (Ed.), *The search for the self* (pp. 737–771). New York: International Universities Press, 1978.

Kohut, H. (1976). Creativeness, charisma and group psychology. In J. E. Gedo & G. H. Pollock (Eds.), *Freud: The fusion of science and humanism. Psychological Issues, 9* [2/3], Monograph 34/35. New York: International Universities Press.

Kohut, H. (1977). *The restoration of the self*. New York: International Universities Press.

Kohut, H. (1978). The disorders of the self and their treatment: An outline. *International Journal of Psycho-Analysis, 59*, 413–425.

Kohut, H. (1979, June). *Four basic definitions of self psychology*. Paper presented to the Workshop on Self Psychology, Chicago, IL.

Kohut, H. (1984). *How does analysis cure?* Chicago: The University of Chicago Press.

Kohut, H., & Wolf, E. (1978). The disorders of the self and their treatment. *International Journal of Psycho-Analysis, 59*, 413–425.

Lachmann, F. M. (1984). Self psychology and psychotherapy: Discussion of "Selfobjects, Development and Psychotherapy" by M. F. Basch, and "Psychoanalytic Psychotherapy: A Contemporary Perspective," by A. Ornstein. In P. Stepansky & A. Goldberg (Eds.), *Kohut's legacy: Contributions to self psychology*. Hillsdale, NJ: Analytic Press.

Lichtenberg, J. (1983). An application of the self psychological viewpoint to psychoanalytic technique. In J. Lichtenberg & S. Kaplan (Eds.), *Reflections on self psychology*. Hillsdale, NJ: The Analytic Press.

Miller, A. (1981). *The drama of the gifted child*. New York: Basic Books.

Muslin, H. (1974). Clinical exercises in empathy. *Diseases of the Nervous System, 6*: 384–387.

Muslin, H. (1984). Empathy and the self/selfobject dyad. *The Hillside Journal of Clinical Psychiatry, 6*, 91–100.

Muslin, H. (1985). Heinz Kohut: Beyond the pleasure principle. Contributions to psychoanalysis. In J. Reppen (Ed.), *Beyond Freud, A study of modern psychoanalytic theorists*. Hillsdale, NJ: Analytic Press.

Muslin, H. (1986). On working through in self psychology. In A. Goldberg (Ed.), *Progress in self psychology*. New York: Analytic Press.

Muslin, H., Burstein, A. G., Gedo, J., & Sadow, L. (1967). Research on the supervisory process. *Archives of General Psychiatry, 16*, 427–431.

Muslin, H., & Gill, M. (1978). Transference in the Dora case. *Journal of the American Psychoanalytic Association, 26*(2), 311–328.

Muslin, H., & Schlessinger, N. (1971). Toward the teaching and learning of empathy. *Bulletin of the Menninger Clinic, 35*(4), 262–271.

Muslin, H., & Val, E. (1980). Supervision and self-esteem in psychiatric teaching. *American Journal of Psychotherapy, 35*(4), 545–555.

Muslin, H. & Val, E. (in press). Supervision: A teaching-learning paradigm. In K. Field, B. Cohler, & G. Wool (Eds.), *Motive and meaning: A psychoanalytic perspective on learning and education*. New York: International Universities Press.

Ornstein, A. (1984). Psychoanalytic psychotherapy: A contemporary perspective. In P. Stepansky & A. Goldberg (Eds.), *Kohut's legacy: Contributions to self psychology*. Hillsdale, NJ: The Analytic Press.

Ornstein, P. H. & Ornstein, A. (1985). Clinical understanding and explaining: The empathic vantage point. In A. Goldberg (Ed.), *Progress in self psychology* (vol. 1, pp. 43–61). New York: Guilford Press.

Palombo, J. (1982). The psychology of the self and the termination of treatment. *Clinical Social Work Journal, 10*, 15–27.

Racker, H. (1957). The meanings and uses of countertransference. *The Psychoanalytic Quarterly, 26*, 303–357.

Racker, H. (1968). *Transference and countertransference*. New York: International Universities Press.

Schlessinger, N., & Robbins, F. (1983). *A developmental view of the psychoanalytic process: Follow-up studies and their consequences*. New York: International Universities Press.

Stepansky, P. & Goldberg, A. (Eds.) (1984). *Kohut's legacy: Contributions to self psychology*. Hillside, NJ: Analytic Press.

Stolorow, R. & Lachmann, F. (1980). *Psychoanalysis of developmental arrests: Theory and treatment*. New York: International Universities Press.

Stone, L. (1961). *The psychoanalytic situation*. New York: International Universities Press.

Tarachow, S. (1963). *An introduction to psychotherapy*. New York: International Universities Press.

Tolpin, M. (1971). On the beginning of a cohesive self. *The Psychoanalytic Study of the Child, 26*, 316–352. New Haven: Yale University Press.

Tolpin, M. (1978). Selfobjects and oedipal objects: A crucial developmental distinction. *The Psychoanalytic Study of the Child, 33*, 167–187. New Haven: Yale University Press.

Tolpin, M. (1983). Corrective emotional experience: A self psychological reevaluation. In A. Goldberg (Ed.), *The future of psychoanalysis*. New York: International Universities Press.

Tolpin, P. (1983). Self psychology and the interpretation of dreams. In A. Goldberg (Ed.), *The future of psychoanalysis*. New York: International Universities Press.

Tower, L. (1956). Countertransference. *Journal of the American Psychoanalytic Association, 4,* 224–255.

Val, E. (1982). Self-esteem, regulation and narcissism. *The Annual of Psychoanalysis, 9,* 221–232.

Val, E., Flaherty, J., & Gaviria, M. (1982). Psychological management of affective disorders. In E. Val, M. Gaviria, & J. Flaherty (Eds.), *Affective disorders: Psychopathology and treatment*. Chicago: Yearbook Medical Publishers.

Val, E., Gaviria, M., & Flaherty, J. (Eds.) (1982). *Affective disorders: Psychopathology and treatment*. Chicago: Yearbook Medical Publishers.

Val, E., & Gaviria, M. (in press). Borderline personality disorders. In J. Flaherty, J. Davis, & R. Chanon (Eds.), *Clinical manual of psychiatric therapeutics*. New York: Appleton-Century-Crofts.

Wallerstein, R. (1986). *Forty-two lives in treatment*. New York: The Guilford Press.

Wolf, E. (1976). Ambience and abstinence. *The Annual of Psychoanalysis, 4,* 101–115.

Wolf E. (1980). On the developmental line of selfobject relations. In A. Goldberg (Ed.), *Advances in self psychology*. New York: International Universities Press.

Wolf, E. (1983). Empathy and countertransference. In A. Goldberg (Ed.), *The future of psychoanalysis*. New York: International Universities Press.

Zetzel, E. R. (1956). Current concepts of transference. *International Journal of Psycho-Analysis, 37,* 369–376.

Index

215